THE
HOLLYWOOD
BODY PLAN

66

To my wife Cara
and sons Bailey,
Beau and Coby.

You are my life force
and inspiration.

99

21 MINUTES FOR 21 DAYS
TO TRANSFORM YOUR BODY FOR LIFE

THE
HOLLYWOOD BODY PLAN

DAVID HIGGINS
PERSONAL TRAINER TO THE STARS

WITH ROSAMUND URWIN

PHOTOGRAPHY BY ANDREW BURTON

CONTENTS

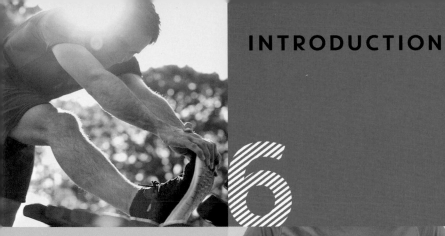
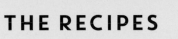
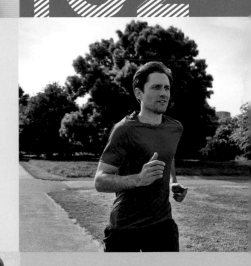
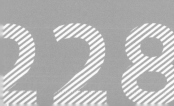

INTRODUCTION

Congratulations! You have taken the first step towards a fitter, healthier, happier you: opening this book. That means you want to feel and look better and you also know you want help to do it. Now let's fix you together.

The human body is amazing – just think of everything it can do (I recommend YouTube videos of the gymnast Simone Biles for evidence of this). It will support you and sustain you if you take care of it.

That's why we should treat it like a temple. Instead, most of us vandalise our bodies. We don't carry out maintenance early enough, instead allowing damage to build up by failing to correct postural problems when they first appear.

Modern life has made it easy to slip into the habit of using your body as nothing more than a vessel – the machine that you're carried around in. That means you stop taking care of yourself physically. But we need our bodies in a good condition if we are going to thrive.

I've been helping people achieve amazing results for 15 years. I will help you identify what is holding you back and show you the changes you need to make to your lifestyle and diet to transform your body. It's about increasing the base level of your fitness so you can live a longer, better life, and about freeing you from pain.

I will get you moving more, but I will also get you moving better. I will show you the kind of exercise that is most beneficial to you and how to treat and prevent the aches and pains that can chip away at your health and happiness. You may eat less than you do now while following my programme but, more importantly, you will eat better. I also want you to start thinking differently about food. My aim is to build the foundations for a healthy future for you – this isn't about developing a 6-pack, but putting the building blocks down to create a healthy lifestyle. I'll give you a framework to follow which will make you understand your body better and make you feel more confident in working out what your body needs in the future.

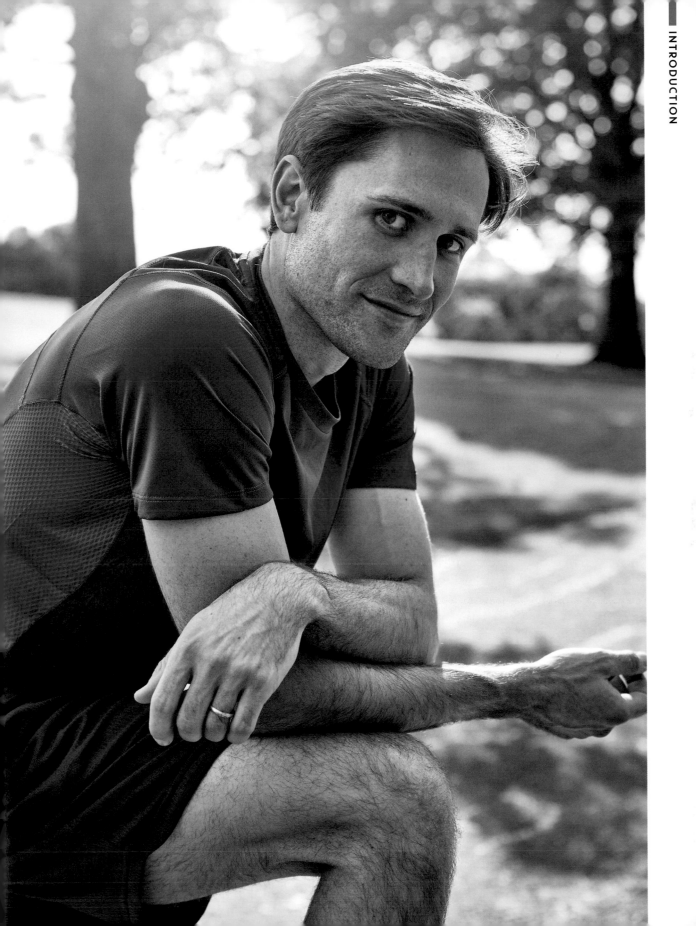

> **I WILL GET YOU MOVING MORE, BUT I WILL ALSO GET YOU MOVING BETTER. I WILL SHOW YOU THE KIND OF EXERCISE THAT IS MOST BENEFICIAL TO YOU AND HOW TO TREAT AND PREVENT THE ACHES AND PAINS THAT CAN CHIP AWAY AT YOUR HEALTH AND HAPPINESS.**

The way we use our bodies now has drifted a long way from how they were designed to be used. We live in a box; we walk around in feet coffins called shoes; we are on our computers and phones constantly; we eat most of the same foods on repeat. And we certainly sit far too much and stand far too little.

Having a desk job can mean you sit for 8 hours at work before going home to collapse on the sofa exhausted in front of the TV. This lifestyle has turned most of us into what I call 'office athletes' – your body has become honed for sitting.

Whether you're running a marathon or sitting in an office for 8 hours a day, your body learns by repetition and will find the most efficient way to hold itself in order to use the minimum amount of energy. Sitting down all day causes you to have a bio-mechanical dysfunction: you'll have tight hips, a weak core (the muscles around your trunk), tight pecs (the muscles in your upper chest), a tight neck and rounded shoulders.

Across the world, backache is the leading cause of disability. And yet it is avoidable. We need to address the underlying causes of the pain and we need to treat them properly when they do occur.

If you're feeling broken – you're dealing with chronic aches or you want a lasting change in the number you see on the scales – this is the book for you.

But it's also the book for you if you're just worried about the path you're currently on. Maybe you look around the office at older colleagues, or you look at your parents, and you don't want to suffer either pain or weight gain like them. This book will show you how to tackle problems early so they don't build up.

Most books say 'do this' but I will also explain *why* you should do this. Some personal trainers take a military approach to fitness and seem to get their kicks out of barking instructions at their clients. That isn't me. I want this book to feel like an arm around your shoulder as you revamp your body and your life. I'm coming on this journey with you.

I want to show you that with only a small time commitment each day, you can stop your body feeling broken. If you have time to binge-watch TV, you definitely have 21 minutes a day to do my exercises.

My Body Dynamix course teaches you how to address aches and niggles – how to release the tight muscles in your neck so you can alleviate pain, for example – but my broader message is that it is possible to reset your entire lifestyle. The Hollywood Body Plan is your chance to hit refresh and overhaul your health – and your life. There's never going to be a better time to start than right now.

There are 3 fundamental parts to the Hollywood Body Plan (*see the programme outlined in full on page 54*).

1. MOVEMENT AND POSTURAL CORRECTION
The inital 21-day Body Reset is a corrective exercise programme that will close the gap between how you currently move and how you should move. It will only take 21 minutes a day and will put you back on the right path physically. Once you have completed the 21-day Body Reset, you graduate to the Transformational Programme, a more dynamic workout.

2. FOOD
For the first 21 days there's a simultaneous nutritional plan (note: I am not calling this a diet!) to match the exercise programme. This book includes the recipes you need to get you back on the right track with your eating.

3. SELF-CARE: THE FOREVER FIX
This will teach you how to address any pain you have yourself. If you have neck pain, backache, or a knee that's causing you grief, this is the book for you. I'm going to build you back up in the best possible way.

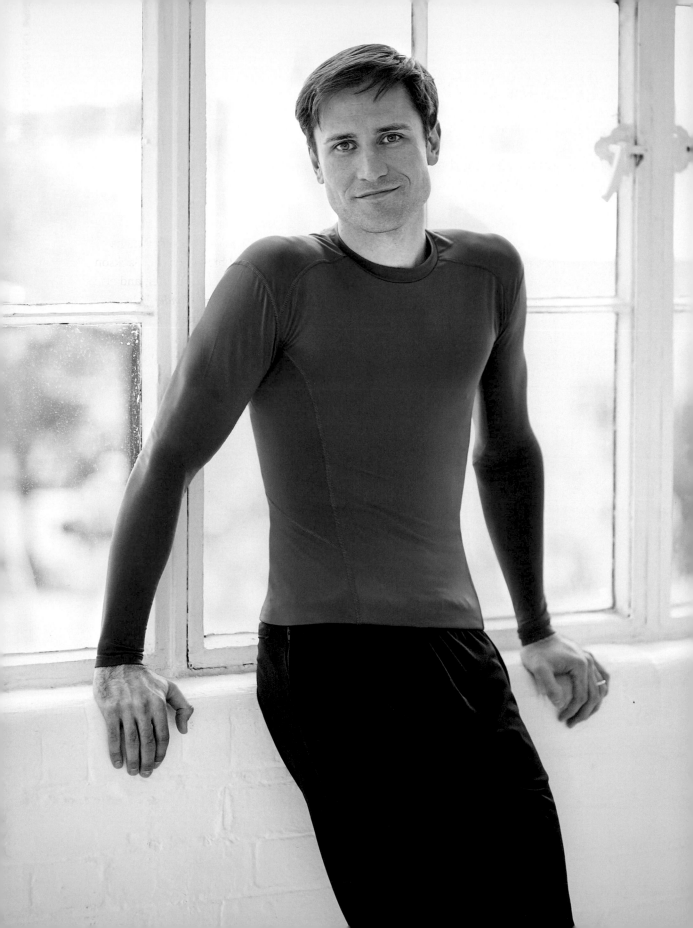

ABOUT ME

I am a personal trainer and physical therapist who now works in the world of film and TV.

My specialism is preparing actors and actresses for film roles, especially those that are physically gruelling. I've worked with Margot Robbie, Samuel L. Jackson and Colin Firth, supermodels like Naomi Campbell and Claudia Schiffer, and also TV presenters such as Nigella Lawson. My film credits include *Wonder Woman*, *Kingsman: The Golden Circle* and *Justice League* (you can sometimes spot my name whizzing by in the credits at the end). My most recent movies include *Mission: Impossible – Fallout* and *Fantastic Beasts and Where to Find Them*. I also co-founded the health and fitness company BodySPace.

I could never have imagined this would be my life. I grew up in Australia and my family didn't have much: if we wanted a snack, we'd take an apple off the tree.

When I was a kid, I remember watching an old man whose spine had collapsed and whose head was out of whack. He was walking at almost 45 degrees. I remember thinking, 'I want to help him move better.' It was a moment that stayed with me.

As a teenager, I began playing Aussie rules football. It took over my life and was my great sporting love. I played at state level for Victoria. When I went to Victoria University in Melbourne to study exercise rehabilitation, I trained 6 days a week and played in a match every Saturday.

But when I was just 19, I was injured after an illegal tackle. I dislocated my shoulder and tore my ribs from my sternum. Doctors told me I was no longer allowed to play contact sport. I was devastated – I couldn't get out of bed for about 6 months. It was the first time I learned how debilitating pain can be.

My life story really isn't a tragedy, though. Eventually, I realised the only way I could motivate myself to carry on was to think about finishing my degree. I remember waking up one morning and trying to put my hands behind my head. I couldn't do it – my injured shoulder was locked – and I thought, 'This has to change. I am too young for this to be happening to me!' I was studying exercise rehabilitation – so it was time for me to rehabilitate myself.

So I learned Pilates on the 'reformer', a piece of exercise equipment that resembles a torture rack and is resistance based. I used it to give myself rehab.

Purely through trial and error, I worked out how my shoulder could be fixed: how well I could move it and how I could keep improving it. This became my fitness workout system, which I have called 'Reformer Dynamix'.

Even now, if I don't do certain exercises, my neck and my back start to seize up. I know what I need to do to mitigate against any potential flare ups, though – and that's what I want to pass on to you. I've never stopped learning, either. Working with clients has taught me even more than my sports science degree did.

After finishing my degree, I moved to London in 2004. When I arrived in the UK, I desperately needed work and I found myself cleaning the exercise machines in a gym for £5 an hour. I was quickly promoted to fitness instructor, then rehab personal trainer and later I became a private personal trainer. My particular specialism was the reformer machine.

It was through my work at the gym that I came to be hired to launch the first class-based Pilates business in the UK. Pilates was great for me, but it wasn't perfect – so I started to pull apart the original teachings and tweak what I didn't agree with.

Two years later, I opened a boutique chain of gyms, physio clinics and Pilates studios, which I've since sold. After that, I set up a consultancy company and worked as a health and fitness expert on films and TV. The way I think about the results people hope to achieve has really changed since I started working in the movie industry.

This led me to develop a new muscle treatment called Body Dynamix (see page 230), which focuses on recovery and works hand in hand with my training approach. The idea is to build not just camera-ready bodies but resilient bodies that can do everything and anything that the director demands of them without getting injured.

So why am I writing this book? I love my job and I love seeing the transformation in my clients so I want to bring the knowledge I have acquired in my 15 years in the industry to a wider audience.

My clients often come to me broken: they have muscle pain, they're stressed and terrified of making it worse by exercising incorrectly. The famous have the same problems as the rest of us.

> **MY 21-DAY BODY RESET PLAN IS A SIMPLE GUIDE WHICH WILL HELP YOU REGAIN CONTROL OF YOUR DYSFUNCTIONAL BODY AND GET YOU BACK TO THE ACTIVE LIFE YOU LOVE.**

Take Samuel L. Jackson. I worked with him on *Kingsman: The Secret Service*, *The Avengers*, *The Legend of Tarzan*, *Miss Peregrine's Home for Peculiar Children* and *Kong: Skull Island*. Here's what he said about working with me: '**When I met David, I was broken physically. He patiently and caringly put me back together. Since then, he has done wonders for motivating me and maintaining my physical health. His combination of strength Pilates, stretching and active release can't be compared to anything I've ever done and the results are nothing short of spectacular.**'

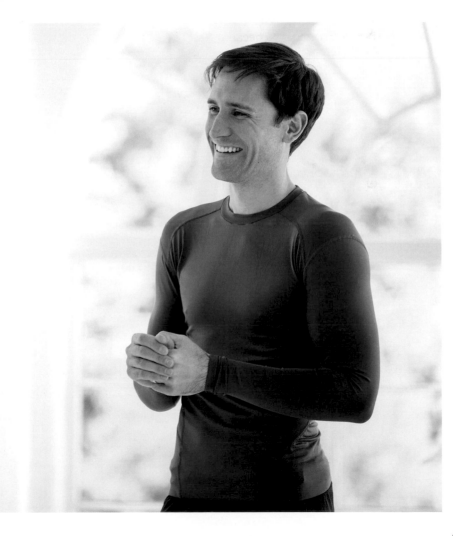

I never enjoyed Pilates until I met David, he transformed me and my opinion and made me look forward to exercising instead of dreading it.

CLAUDIA SCHIFFER

His unique approach taught me to be conscious of my posture and to control my movement so as to maximise strength and ability. I have incorporated David's methods into my daily routine and they continue to deliver results I'd never believed possible.

COLIN FIRTH

FIND YOUR MOTIVATION

You need a motivator, a reason to convince you to get fit or lose weight.
It has to be powerful enough to be a catalyst for behavioural change.
Put a label on why you want to be different. Good intentions alone won't
necessarily work. These are a few possibilities, but really think about
what is the driver for you.

01/
GET YOUR OLD LIFE BACK – THE EPIPHANY MOMENT

Maybe you've had a moment when you thought, 'I want to play with my kids but my back is
messed up' or 'I just can't run around like I used to.' Or maybe it was 'That's enough – I finally
need to lose this baby weight' or 'I want to break the cycle of yo-yo dieting once and for all.'
Perhaps there was a particular moment that you can focus on: finding you were too unfit to
climb the stairs at work without panting, or needing to buy a new wardrobe of bigger clothes.

02/
FIXING AN INJURY

Perhaps, like me, you've had an injury and your physical capabilities changed in an
instant. Or perhaps it is just aches and pains that have arisen through your general lifestyle
– your neck hurts from slumping at a computer all day, say. It takes 10 years of moving
the wrong way to turn that into an injury.

03/
PREVENTION

Your motivation could also be about preventing future damage. Perhaps you have an
elderly relative with a hump back (a dowager's hump); or you have older friends who are
reliant on pain medication to combat chronically sore backs.

04/

IMPROVING HOW YOU RELATE TO YOUR BODY

Think of exercise as a pivot point to take control of yourself physically and to change how you relate to your body. Your movements throughout the day are going to be the major driver of that. My programme retrains your every movement, so you can move your body without hurting it.

05/

BOOSTING YOUR MOOD

Exercise releases endorphins so it isn't just good for your physical health – it gives psychological and even social benefits. Ever heard of 'runners' high'? That's endorphins. On top of that, regular exercise will reduce your stress levels. You can sweat out stress, essentially. It also helps combat insomnia, improving your sleep quality and making it easier for you to get out of bed in the morning. It can even ease anxiety – the instant boost from getting moving can translate into a more long-term comfort.

Exercise is the best route to a healthier lifestyle – and it will also make you happier.

06/

LIFE MILESTONE

Your motivation may even be an important birthday or a new year's resolution – this is the year that you will get really fit. It may not feel like it, but finding this motivator is a vital first step. Think of it as the positive equivalent of a mid-life crisis. You needed this epiphany to jolt you into thinking, 'I really need to start looking after myself.' This is the time to say, 'I've got nothing to lose – besides my beer gut or my baby weight.'

Don't beat yourself up for gaining weight or for not looking after yourself better in the past – guilt won't help. Instead, feel proud of yourself for deciding to make a change now.

NEXT STEPS

Now that you know what your motivation is, start sharing it:

WRITE DOWN A COMMITMENT TO YOURSELF THAT YOU CAN RE-READ LATER (PARTICULARLY IN THE MOMENTS WHEN THIS PROGRAMME FEELS HARD) AND SHOW THIS STATEMENT TO PEOPLE CLOSE TO YOU.

TELL YOUR FRIENDS AND FAMILY, 'I AM GOING TO GET FIT AND LOOK AFTER MYSELF BETTER.' A COMMITMENT FEELS STRONGER AFTER YOU DISCUSS IT WITH THOSE CLOSE TO YOU. THIS JOURNEY WILL BE EASIER IF YOU HAVE SUPPORTIVE FRIENDS AND FAMILY TO HELP KEEP YOU ON TRACK.

STICK A NOTE TO YOURSELF ON THE FRIDGE, REMINDING YOURSELF WHY YOU ARE DOING THIS.

UPLOAD A VIDEO TO OUR FACEBOOK PAGE FACEBOOK.COM/DAVIDHIGGINSLONDON WHERE YOU CAN TALK ABOUT WHY YOU WANT TO CHANGE.

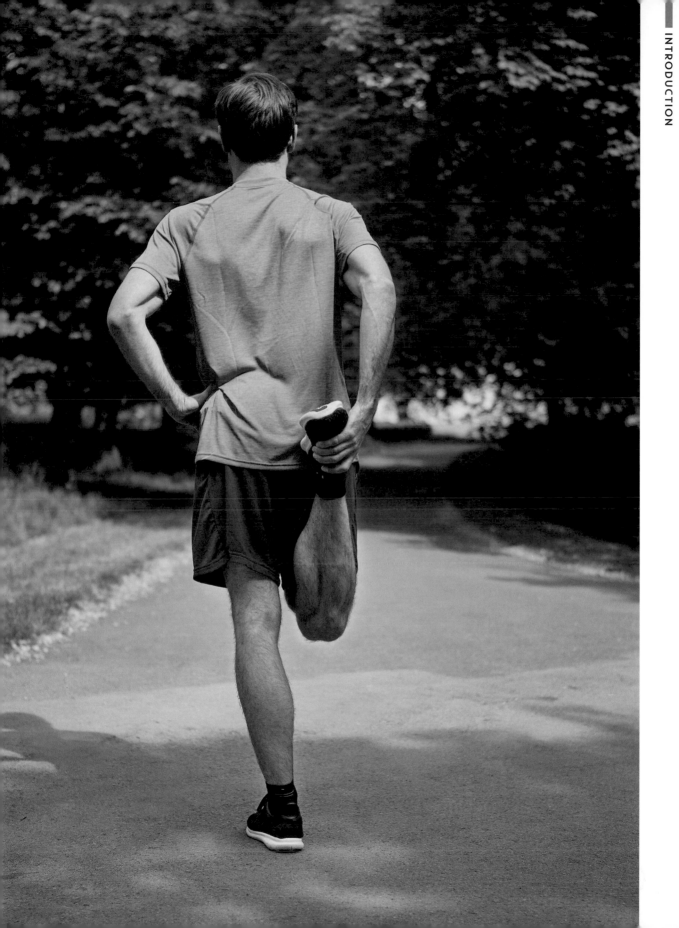

CHANGE HOW YOU THINK ABOUT TIME

There are two versions of yourself: your present self (who you are right now) and your future self (who you want to be). Most of us are terrible at thinking about our future selves – the one who wants to be healthier, thinner, fitter. We instead focus on our present selves – the one who wants instant gratification. Our present selves tend to want quick fixes – but worthwhile, meaningful change takes time.

While crash diets don't work, you can actually reverse degeneration quite quickly. Think about it like this: you may have had 20 years of eating poorly and moving in a harmful way, but within just 12 months – a 20th of that time – you can address it all. That's actually fast.

People always ask, 'How long will it take for me to lose weight?' and 'How long will it take for me to get fit?' The better question to ask, though, is 'How long did it take for me to get to the position I'm in now?' And then just remember that it will take less time to fix it – but it won't be instant.

With food, it isn't as simple as calories in and calories out – that is an old-school approach to healthy eating. It's also about the quality of the food being eaten, the timing of meals, and the body's hormonal response to food. You should be aiming for a healthy, sustainable way to reduce your weight – not a quick fix. That said, if you were to drop your calorific intake by just 10 per cent – and increase the proportion of calories that come from vegetables – that would lead to a healthy, slow weight loss.

66

DON'T BEAT YOURSELF UP FOR GAINING WEIGHT OR FOR NOT LOOKING AFTER YOURSELF BETTER IN THE PAST – GUILT WON'T HELP. INSTEAD, FEEL PROUD OF YOURSELF FOR DECIDING TO MAKE A CHANGE NOW.

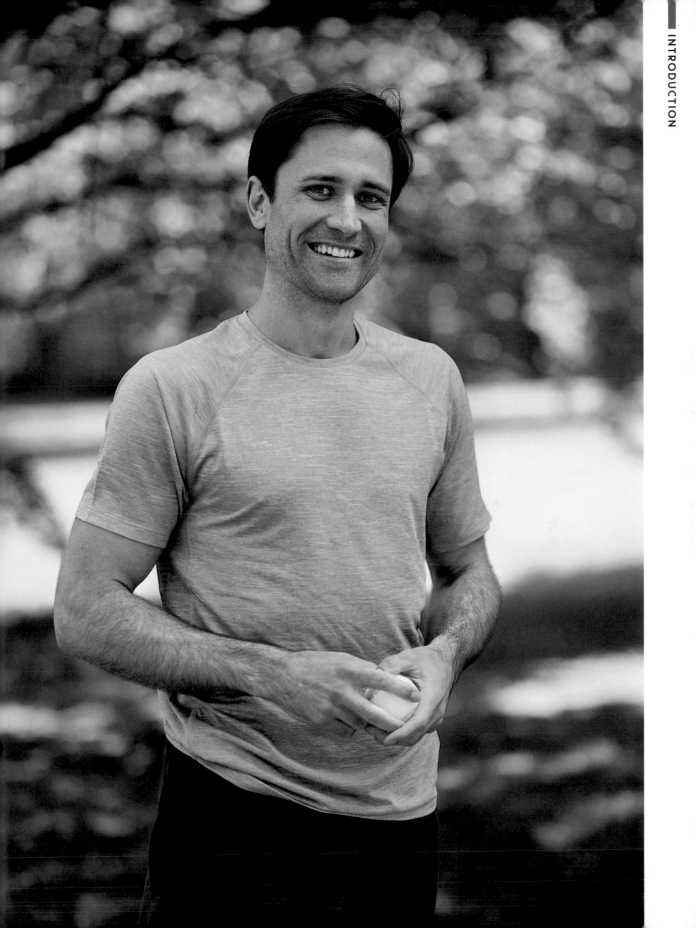

WHAT'S STANDING IN YOUR WAY?

01/
INERTIA

I often hear people with good intentions make the mistake of saying, 'I've got to lose some weight before I get fit.' Why? They work together, they are two halves of one whole. You can do them in tandem: get moving and simultaneously think more about what goes in your mouth. Taking a two-pronged approach is much more likely to be successful, not just because you are both expending extra energy by exercising and consuming fewer calories by eating more healthily, but because you won't want to undermine the benefits of moving more by chowing down on a chocolate bar.

When it comes to exercise and tackling the problems that build up in our bodies as a result of our sedentary lifestyles, sometimes people are also scared to make a first step, because they say they don't want to upset the balance that they have going in case it gets worse. But it will get worse if you just keep carrying on. It'll get worse because you're not doing anything to fix it.

02/
BODY BAGGAGE

People carry a lot of 'body baggage' – mostly past injuries that they're paranoid about. I hear it the whole time as a personal trainer – 'When I was 11, I broke my arm' or 'When I was 25, I did in my knee running' and that person might be 40 now. That decades-old injury doesn't have anything to do with anything any more. It would be much better to let go of it, than to obsess about it.

One of the most common things I hear is, 'I can't run because my knees hurt.' It's actually more complicated than that. Your knees hurt because your glutes aren't working properly and your back is messed up. It's not that you can't run – it's probably that some fitness or medical professional has told you not to run because it will exacerbate the problem and they don't want to deal with it. They're kicking it into the long grass, when really what you need to do is sort yourself out so you *can* run. That's what this book will help you with.

03/
STRESS

Modern life is really stressful. Stress is both an everyday feeling for so many of us and a major obstacle when it comes to changing our lives. Perhaps you feel, 'I can't possibly make time to look after myself because I've got too much to do.' I know it can feel like that. It never seems like there are enough hours in the day. What with work, family, friends, the housework, and hopefully squeezing in some down time, it's not surprising that many of us think that trying to fit in exercise would be impossible.

But it's like the fact that you need to put on your own life vest before you put on your child's – in order to look after other people, you have to look after yourself first. It's easy to forget that.

If you're juggling family commitments as well as work, it's hard to give much attention to your own health, but spending some time on yourself will actually help everyone around you. You will be more efficient at work and in the home by taking care of your body.

Stress is a form of fear. Whatever emotion you are feeling, your posture will reflect it. So when you're happy, you'll find yourself in open, confident poses; if you're scared and stressed, you'll shrink yourself with your posture, as though to protect your vital organs. Unfortunately, stress comes hand-in-hand with the easiest way to hold ourselves at our desks. So you get a perfect storm of bad posture and stress adding to the tension in your back.

Psychological stresses can often manifest themselves physically as well. When you're stressed, you hold tension in your neck or in your back. That means you start to 'round' your shoulders, hunching them, and that will lead to neck problems. It is all inter-connected. Even how you breathe will be affected by stress.

Your neck is one of the most common spots in the body to be afflicted. Stress can both trigger a problem and make it more severe – the initial neck pain might be caused by a muscle injury, but stress extends the pain.

> **"**
> **IF YOU'RE JUGGLING FAMILY COMMITMENTS AS WELL AS WORK, IT'S HARD TO GIVE MUCH ATTENTION TO YOUR OWN HEALTH, BUT SPENDING SOME TIME ON YOURSELF WILL ACTUALLY HELP EVERYONE AROUND YOU.**

23

AGE

In the past, we saw age as an excuse for letting our health and fitness slip away – we thought that the passing years brought inevitable decline. Certainly, getting older presents challenges. When I was a teenager, I ate whatever I liked; now I have to be much more conscious of what is going in my mouth. That was an unwelcome change that arrived around the time of my 30th birthday.

But, that said, every extra candle on the cake doesn't have to make us less fit. A focused programme benefits ageing athletes as much as the young. Much of the decline that we think goes hand-in-hand with ageing can actually be blamed on a sedentary lifestyle; studies show that those who continue to train and even compete athletically are much less likely to suffer from the ailments we consider age-induced.

Just think of all those celebrities – George Clooney, Sandra Bullock, Brad Pitt – who have stayed just as fit in their 40s and 50s as they were in their 20s. Patrick Stewart had a 6-pack aged 75! So you should set yourself the same fitness goals as you did when you were younger.

One particularly common myth is that you shouldn't start running as you get older or you'll destroy your knees. Of course, running isn't for everyone but there are plenty of studies that have now debunked the idea that it will universally cause harm. It depends much more on your biomechanics than on how old you are. Running is a good form of exercise for most people, but resistance-based training is even more important as you get older – especially at certain times in your life, like if you're a woman going through the menopause.

It's never too late to get fitter. Age is not an insurmountable barrier.

> **I WANT TO SHOW YOU THAT WITH ONLY A SMALL COMMITMENT EACH DAY, YOU CAN STOP YOUR BODY FEELING BROKEN. IF YOU HAVE TIME TO BINGE-WATCH TV, YOU DEFINITELY HAVE 21 MINUTES A DAY TO DO MY EXERCISES.**

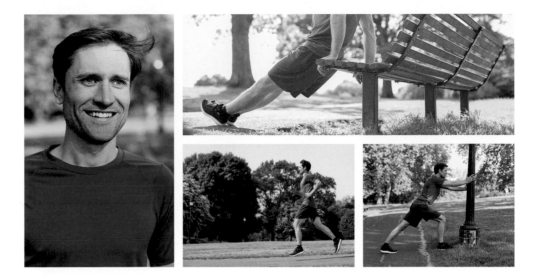

05/

LIFE GETS IN THE WAY

As you get older, though, life usually becomes more complicated, too. You may have growing commitments – marriage, kids, mortgages or high rent bills, a more demanding job, older relatives to care for – and it can feel like your health has run away from you. It falls down the pecking order as the stresses and responsibilities (and joys!) in the rest of your life grow.

I'm a father of 3 and that has certainly changed my perspective. Keeping fit isn't so much about looking good now, it's about being an active dad and giving myself the best chance of being an active grandad one day, too.

I can also see my parents getting older and I'm starting to think about how they'll be cared for. It has given me a fresh perspective – we all tend to think our parents are superhuman when we're growing up. Seeing them as vulnerable is hard.

What both having children and watching my parents get older has brought home to me is that health is wealth. You find it's the trivial-sounding incidents that screw with you when you're older: the falls, the trips, the bangs and bumps.

If you do have kids or other caring responsibilities, it often means you put your interests at the bottom of the list. Don't relegate your own needs to the bottom of the pile. Don't think that taking time for yourself – to exercise or make a proper meal – is selfish. By investing time in yourself, you will be much more able to care for your family well.

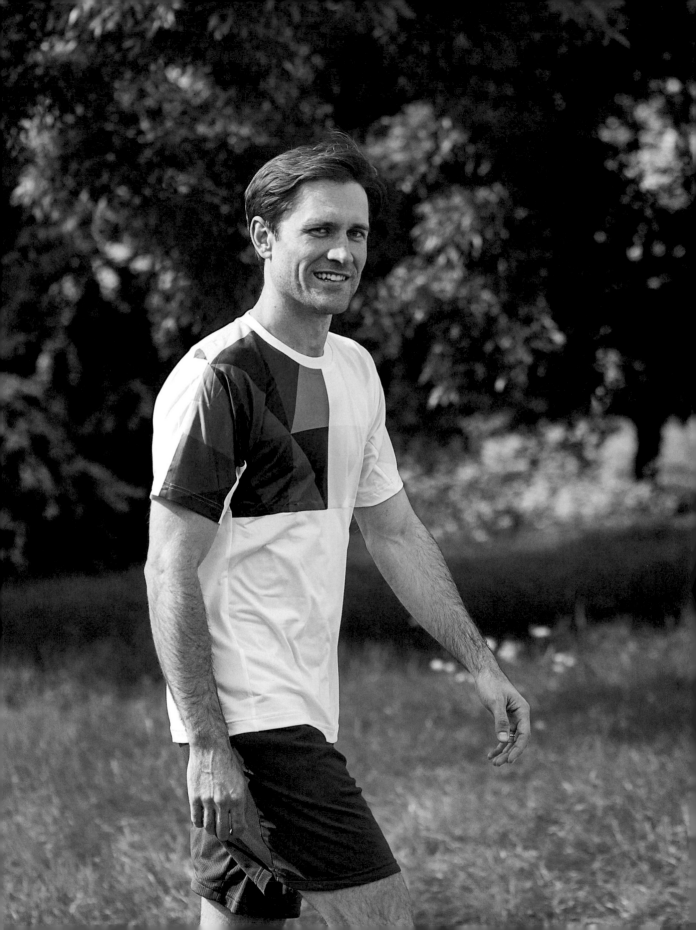

GIVING YOURSELF A TARGET

It is really important that you give yourself a target to aim for. Think of it as a journey: you need to know where you're going, as well as the path you're taking.

This target has to be achievable. Here are a few suggestions for inspiration:

 RUNNING A 10K OR COMPLETING THE 3 PEAKS CHALLENGE

 BECOMING PAIN FREE BY A CERTAIN BIRTHDAY

 WEARING BEACH CLOTHES THIS SUMMER

 LOWERING YOUR CHOLESTEROL

 NOT FEELING LIKE YOU HAVE TO BREATHE IN TO HOLD IN YOUR STOMACH FOR PHOTOS!

 NOT MINDING WHEN YOU SEE YOURSELF IN CHANGING ROOM MIRRORS

 FITTING INTO THE SKINNY JEANS THAT ARE CURRENTLY LURKING AT THE BACK OF YOUR WARDROBE

FIRST PRINCIPLES

You need to get back to basics to heal yourself. You might think the things I am about to explain – how to breathe, how to walk, how to sleep, how to sit – are so basic that you can skip this part.

I get where you're coming from. If you didn't know how to breathe, you would be dead. If you didn't know how to sleep, you would start to fall apart, both physically and mentally. And most of us are lucky enough to be able to stand, walk and sit.

But that doesn't mean you're doing it perfectly. In fact, for basic functions that we have to do every single day, we're not terribly good at any of this.

So please do read what follows.

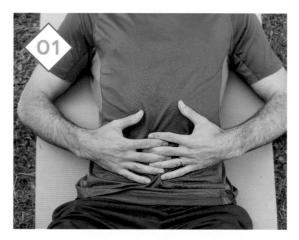

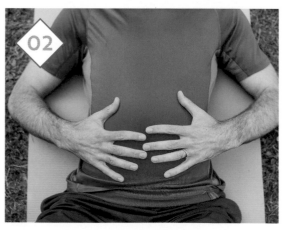

HOW TO BREATHE

You want to breathe like a baby, which means from the belly. This is also called 'conscious breathing' and is the optimal way to breathe for your body.

To test you are doing it correctly:

01. Lie down on your back and place your hands on your rib cage with your fingers interlocked.

02. When you breathe in, your fingers should come away from each other.

This is the way we were supposed to breathe, before our bodies adapted to the poisonous combination of a high-stress lifestyle and chronic stillness. People with good posture tend to breathe better, too.

WHY IS CONSCIOUS BREATHING SO IMPORTANT?

Dysfunctional or improper breathing habits affect our brain, heart and muscle function. With less oxygen in the system, your muscles will not perform at their optimal level. It will also significantly impede recovery.

FOUR BREATHING PRINCIPLES

01. Use your nose – it is nature's air cleaner. If you breathe in and out through your nose, the air is filtered, meaning what reaches your lungs has some of the problematic particles removed. Your nose also warms and moistens the air before it reaches the lungs.

02. Breathe with your belly. About 70–80 per cent of every breath should be controlled by your belly (diaphragm). The rest should be supported by your abdomen, neck and shoulder muscles. Unfortunately, poor posture means about 70–80 per cent of each breath is performed by our neck and shoulder muscles. That's partly why our neck gets sore after a long day in front of a computer.

03. Relax your breath. Our breathing reflects our thoughts, feelings and our physical body. If we are anxious, our breath shortens, which reduces the oxygen supply to the brain, which in turn makes the body even more stressed. As we take back control of our breathing, we in turn take back control of our body and our mind.

04. Increase your exhale. The optimal breathing rhythm when you're not exercising is to inhale for 2–3 seconds and exhale for 3–4 seconds, followed by a 2–3 second pause.

POSTURE & RHYTHMIC BREATHING EXERCISE

To reset your breathing, do this as often as you like during the day:
• Breathe in for 5 seconds.
• Hold for 5 seconds.
• Breathe out for 5 seconds.
• Hold for 5 seconds.
• Do this for a minimum of 6 repetitions.
This will help you recalibrate your breathing patterns, reset your posture into an upright, aligned position and improve your awareness of your breath.

HOW TO MOVE

If someone is really broken and they've forgotten how to move, I start them on the floor. That's where we started when we were babies, after all. You have to earn the right to stand up again. It's the old, 'You have to walk before you can run.'

My exercises start you on the floor but if you are really stiff, use my Floor Play Reboot first. It's a 3-minute trick to reset the way you move – like hitting ctrl + alt + del on your PC. It is a great hack to use in the morning after you wake up but you can also do this as often as you like throughout the day, whenever you have 3 minutes and some space to roll around.

FLOOR PLAY REBOOT

01. Lie down on the floor, face down, arms outstretched above your head. Keep your chin tucked in.

02. Roll over on to your back, making sure that your right arm leads the movement, opening the chest; your hips, torso and legs should follow after.

03. Now that you are on your back, slowly lift and bend your left knee. Roll it across your body, allowing the hips to roll you over to return to the start position.

04. Now do this again except leading with your left arm. Once on your back, continue the roll by lifting and bending your right knee, rolling yourself over.

Do this body roll 3–5 times, going back and forth on the floor – this should take 50 seconds.

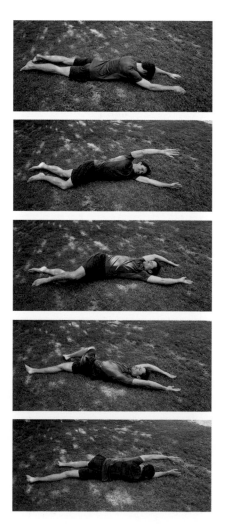

05. Move into a slow Cat Stretch (see page 80) – this should take 20 seconds in each position.

06. Now move into a Pigeon Stretch (see page 64) – 20 seconds on each side.

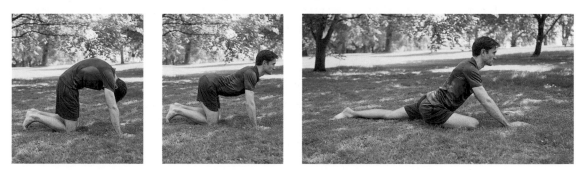

07. Complete a Hip Flexor Stretch (see page 71) with a 20-second reach on each side.

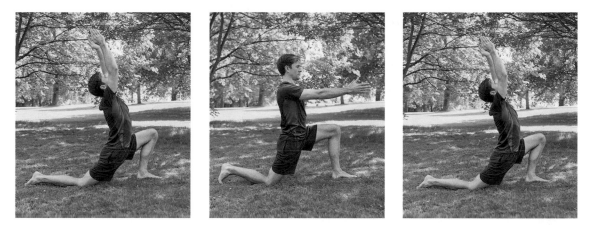

08. Get on to all fours and rock your body weight forward and backward for 20 seconds.

09. Finish in Child's Pose (see page 94) and hold for 10 seconds.

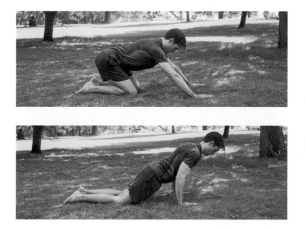

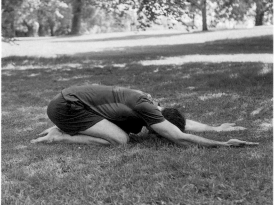

HOW TO WALK

When I walk, with every step I take, I make sure I am grounding my feet. That means gripping the floor with my toes, making sure my knees are slightly externally rotated, my glutes (the muscles in my bottom) are on, my abdominals (the muscles in my stomach) are engaged and my shoulders are back. That might sound like a lot to think about but it is worth it. Most people walk mindlessly – we think it is a natural movement because we've done it so long so we don't think about what we're doing.

01. The common mistakes you might be making include turning your feet out and collapsing at the ankles, so your knees rotate inwards. This is why I see a lot of knee and hip issues.

02. To compensate for that, your hips tilt forward and your leg internally rotates. You end up disengaging the muscles in your stomach (your abdominals) and in your bottom (your glutes), rounding your back and your head starts to poke forward. That's just from not gripping the ground properly.

03. When you walk, you need your heel to strike so you are going more towards the outside border of your foot and you're not going inwards on the arch. Grip and plant the big toe (the little toes will follow) and then push off from there. This shifts the knee out a bit, which encourages your glutes to turn on and do their job of helping support your lower back, knee and foot.

When you are stiff, sore or in pain, you shorten your stride to stop yourself falling over, so essentially you're shuffling. This actually makes you more unstable. When you're in pain you should actually be taking longer strides, because when you have momentum going forward, you are far more stable.

SHOES ARE AWFUL – they stop your feet from moving, which immobilises your arches. So when you do the exercises in the book, please do not wear shoes.

The toes grip the ground
promoting the natural
arch of the foot.

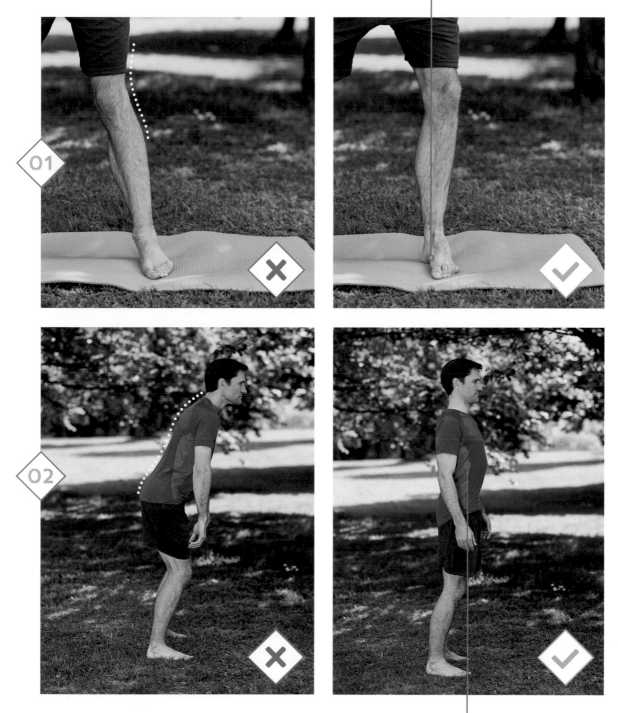

01

02

Neutral position.

HOW TO SIT

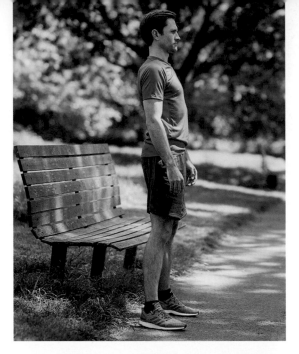

Ideally, we would all sit down a lot less. In fact, we should probably stop sitting at all. But that's not very realistic. So, as mad as this might sound, it's a good idea to assess how you sit. Either enlist the help of a friend or set up a camera so you can get a side profile of yourself. Close your eyes and relax into your regular seated position (don't pretend you always sit up – you don't!).

If you are pulling your shoulders forward, you need to release your chest and your neck. When your mum told you to 'sit up straight', she was on to something: your shoulders need to be pulled back and down.

WHEN YOU SIT DOWN, FOLLOW THESE RULES:

Separate your feet so they are shoulder width apart. Hinge forward at the hips and don't round your spine as you go to sit down.

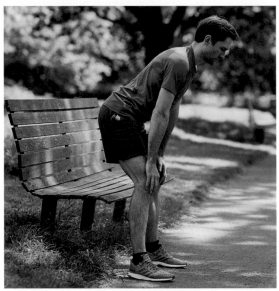

Finally, put your hands on your knees to stabilise yourself as you settle into position.

To stand back up, position your feet wider than your hips, put your hands on your knees and push down as you get back up.

WHAT NOT TO DO:
Twist and bend with your feet together (usually accompanied by a sigh as your bottom hits the seat). This exacerbates everything you are doing wrong.

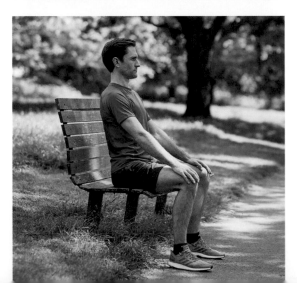

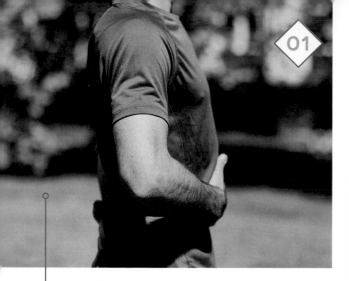

This is called anterior pelvic tilt. This position places excess load on the lower back, which leads to back pain. The muscles in your lower back are overworked and the muscles in front can't do their job.

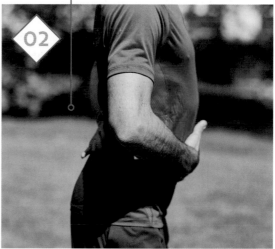

This is what a neutral position looks like. There is equal muscle tone through the stomach at the front and the bottom and spine at the back.

HOW TO RESET YOUR SPINE POSITION

This is something to do throughout the day and also when you are doing my exercise programme so that eventually it becomes your new way of holding yourself – your new normal. You should put little reminders to yourself to do this as often as every hour.

01. Place the back of one hand on your lower back and the other on your stomach.

02. Tilt your hips, so your lower back exaggerates its curve, as though you are trying to push your bottom out.

03. Tilt your hips in the opposite direction.

04. Repeat 4 times.

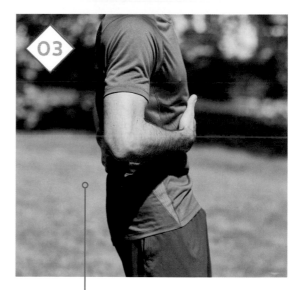

This is called posterior pelvic tilt. This position causes lower back pain because the muscles in front are too tight, which doesn't allow the muscles at the back to do their job.

35

HOW TO SLEEP

When we get tired, we tend to overeat to help us stay alert. And it is rarely carrot sticks and houmous we choose – it's much more likely that we tuck into sugary biscuits or carb-heavy foods. You're not eating because you're hungry but in a bid to keep your eyes open. That's why it's such a good idea to look closely at your sleeping patterns.

Obviously, if you are suffering from severe and protracted insomnia (more than a month of struggling to sleep), please go and see a doctor. But here are 7 tips to help you sleep if the struggle is an intermittent one.

SLEEP FIXES

CREATE A BEDTIME RITUAL

Use the last period before you go to bed as wind-down time – read a novel, have a bath, meditate. Build a barrier that demarcates your active hours from your hours of rest.

BUY AN OLD-FASHIONED ALARM CLOCK

Buy a retro alarm clock so you don't need your phone by your bed and you won't be tempted to check it in the night.

CUT YOUR CAFFEINE INTAKE

This is especially important in the hours before bed. It isn't just coffee that keeps you awake – tea, chocolate and any caffeinated drinks are best avoided. Some painkillers also contain caffeine.

KEEP ELECTRONIC DEVICES OUT OF THE BEDROOM

The blue light your phone or tablet emits will stop you dozing off because it affects levels of the sleep-inducing hormone melatonin. Make sure TVs, computers and other blue-light sources are either entirely off or, better, out of the bedroom completely. Never email or text in bed.

THE MUSCLE CLENCH

Here's a trick that seems to work for a lot of people who are struggling to drop off:

01. As you lie in bed, clench all your muscles as hard as you can.

02. Then slowly release them simultaneously.

The theory is that you may not realise where you are holding tension in your body, and this is a way to release it all.

LAVENDER DREAMS

You may find essential oils help you sleep. Lavender is a classic sleep aid – give some lavender oil a good sniff and it may also help you clear your mind.

PIMP YOUR BED

If you have the money to splash out, it's worth spending it on your bed. Think of it like this: there is almost nowhere that you spend more time.

ASK YOURSELF

01/

ARE YOU GETTING AS MUCH SLEEP AS YOU NEED?

You'll know the signs if the answer is 'no'. Maybe you drift off at your desk, or on your way home. Maybe you have aubergine rings under your eyes. Perhaps you find yourself panicking when you do get to bed about how soon you'll have to wake up.

02/

ARE YOU RELYING ON PRESCRIPTION MEDICATION TO MAKE YOU DRIFT OFF?

This may be little comfort to you, but you're not alone if the answer is yes. In fact, in 2017, the NHS spent around £72m on sleeping pills. The bad news is that, according to recent research, they are not as effective as we imagine them to be. But the issue is bigger – even if they do make you conk out, it may not be the right form of rest. If you go to sleep having taken a sleeping pill, the shuteye you get will be less restorative than natural sleep. That's because these drugs sedate you, rather than putting you to normal sleep. Experts now think the best way to tackle sleeplessness is to deal with the psychological causes.

03/

DO YOU HAVE RHYTHM?

No, I don't mean can you dance, but whether your days stick to the same pattern. This isn't possible for everyone but if you can, try to go to sleep and wake up at the same time every day, even at the weekend.

04/

ARE YOU THE RIGHT TEMPERATURE IN BED?

We have all tossed and turned when we're too hot in bed, or we've woken up shivering when we're too cold. Fiddle with your central heating in the winter or buy a fan for the summer. Just make sure you're creating an environment conducive to sleep – a Goldilocks bedroom, not too hot, not too cold, but just right. The preferred sleep temperature for most people is around 20 degrees centigrade.

05/

ARE YOU PAIN FREE?

One of the big hurdles to sleep – especially as you get older – is pain. It may not be enough to keep you up at night, but it can still stop you entering the deepest stages of sleep. If you are suffering from back pain, try a pillow between your legs. If you are waking up with a stiff neck, check your pillow. If it is too thin or too broad and you sleep on your back, find another one.

06/

IS YOUR ROOM DARK ENOUGH AND QUIET ENOUGH?

Some people need blackness, others silence – work out what your waking triggers are and see if you can find ways to combat them, whether that is blackout curtains or a white noise machine. You could try wearing an eye mask or putting in ear plugs. Some people want the opposite: absolute darkness scares them, or they find themselves drifting off faster when they listen to music. Best to experiment.

HOW TO EAT
8 FOOD RULES TO LIVE BY

01/
VARIETY IS KEY

We hear a lot about 'superfoods' – kale, spinach, seaweed, spirulina and now pineapple – but rather than focusing on eating one particular type of food, try to eat a range of different ones. A simple way of trying to get a wide range of vitamins and minerals is to make sure you are 'seeing the rainbow on your plate'.

RED: The antioxidant lycopene gives tomatoes their red colour and there is some evidence to suggest that lycopene can help reduce blood pressure and cholesterol.

ORANGE/YELLOW: Beta-carotene is what makes fruit and veg such as carrots and squash, orange and yellow. It is turned into vitamin A (good for eye health) in the body.

GREEN: Green fruit and veg get their colour from the pigment chlorophyll, and green vegetables like kale, broccoli and pak choi are good sources of sulforaphane, which studies, including one by the Johns Hopkins University School of Medicine, suggest may help protect against some cancers.

BLUE/PURPLE: Blue and purple fruits such as aubergines, red cabbage and blackberries take their colour from anthocyanins, potent antioxidants that are believed to help protect cells from damage.

02/
EAT LESS MEAT

We eat too much meat and too few vegetables. There's a simple solution: switch it around. Make vegetables the centre of two of your meals a day and you'll look and feel far better.

03/
DRINK MORE WATER

Our bodies can absorb and break down nutrients in food – and that includes the water in food. However, drinking water can help you lose weight by making you feel more full.

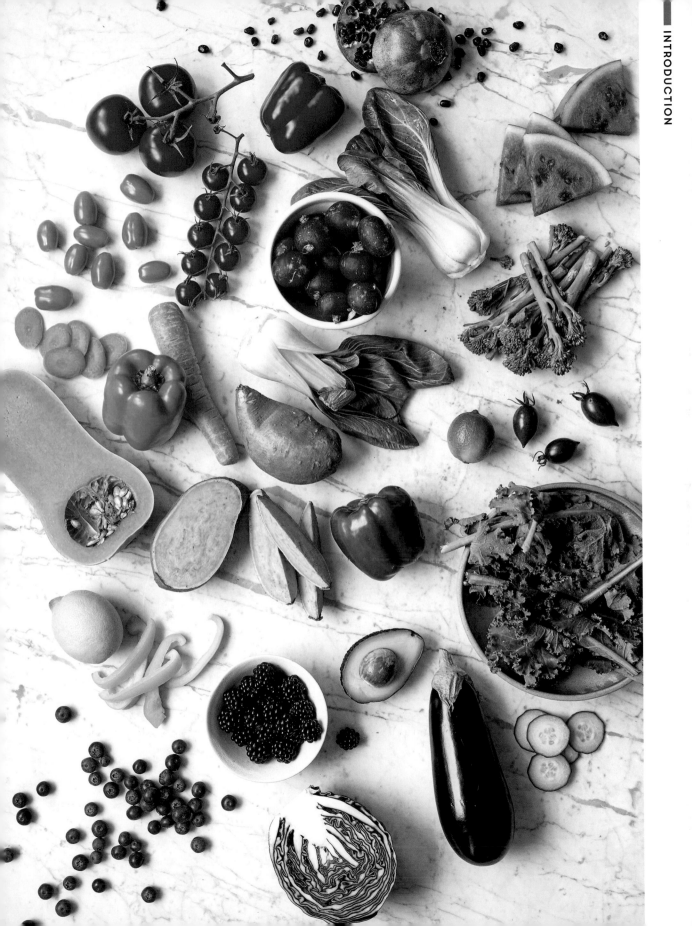

DITCH THE FRIED FOOD AND CUT DOWN ON SUGARY TREATS AND PROCESSED FOOD

Every time food manufacturers modify processed food, they seem to create a new problem. For example, low-fat foods used to be heralded as healthier alternatives but while they may have less fat, they are often very high in sugar. Both processed and fried foods are often packed with unhealthy fats. Regularly eating foods that are fried in unhealthy oils has been shown to put you at a higher risk of developing heart disease and diabetes and becoming obese. The main problems are commercially fried foods but processed food can also be high in a spectrum of nasties, including sugar, high fructose corn syrup and artificial ingredients.

Don't use sugar to reward yourself. That's a behaviour deep-rooted in childhood. It means we have come to associate sugar with comfort and joy.

05/

REDUCE YOUR PORTION SIZE

There's a study that neatly illustrates the dangers of the family-sized bag of chocolates. Back in 2000, a team of researchers led by Brian Wansink, the scientist in charge of Cornell University's Food and Brand Lab, went to the cinema and gave some punters a free bucket of popcorn and asked them to answer questions after the movie. What the study was actually looking into was irrational eating behaviour. Essentially, whether we keep chowing down even when we're not enjoying it.

Because this wasn't lick-your-fingers buttery and delicious popcorn – it was off. Rank. And yet, that didn't stop people eating it! But the test wasn't just looking at whether they ate it. Some of the participants were given popcorn in a medium-sized tub, the rest were given a large bucket. Would those with bigger buckets eat more? Yes. A lot more. On average, they ate 53 per cent more popcorn than those with the medium buckets. That translated as about 21 extra handfuls of popcorn and 173 more calories. The researchers have repeated this study elsewhere with the same results.

So what does this tell us? Something simple, yet radical. When we pile more on our plate – even if we don't really want it – we eat more. So, you can trick yourself into eating less by swapping a dinner plate for a salad plate. Use your smallest bowls. Drink out of wine glasses, not giant goblets. And don't eat snack food directly out of the bag or box – instead put a portion on to a plate.

06/

CUT OUT ALCOHOL

When you're doing the 21-day programme, go alcohol cold turkey. It's only 21 days! Once the programme is over, you can have wine again. But there are reasons to cut down even once the 21 days are up. Alcohol makes you worse at exercise, it can make you more anxious and impair your judgement. Drinking heavily is linked to obesity, it irks the gut, has a dehydrating effect and, obviously, can give you a thumping headache in the morning. Alcohol also inhibits control – many of us overeat after drinking and so the morning-after regret isn't always just a sore head, it's also about those unhealthy foods we ate.

For the 21 days, also avoid energy drinks and carbonated drinks. You can drink coffee and tea, just don't add sugar or sweeteners, and limit caffeinated drinks to 3 a day.

07/

TRY A PROBIOTIC FIRST THING IN THE MORNING

This is anecdotal, but probiotics have certainly helped me. I only started taking one after a gut trauma. I had a horrific bout of food poisoning on an aeroplane in 2016 and found that, afterwards, I would often feel bloated and I had a distended belly. I started doing some research into how best to fix my gut and that's when I stumbled upon an English company called Symprove. Their probiotic sorted me out. A farmer developed it. I can't say it's delicious, but it keeps me feeling well. There have been independent clinical trials that show that probiotics help sufferers of IBS.

08/

STOP WOLFING DOWN YOUR FOOD

When you eat really fast, you don't give your brain time to register the signals from your stomach telling you that you are full. A number of studies have shown that slower eaters are sometimes thinner. So chew your food more before swallowing – chew each mouthful at least 10 times. Think about it as getting more bang for your buck from your food.

This is also why you should try to avoid eating at your desk at work. In that environment, of course you're going to eat rapidly. So, whenever possible, step away from the desk, find somewhere to sit down and try to take at least half an hour over lunch.

41

SO ... GET STARTED!

My 21-day Body Reset Programme will prepare you for lasting change in your life. It will reboot your system. This programme is for everybody – it's not just for someone who has an injury or has never exercised, nor is it just for people who are postnatal, although it is for all of those people. It is for anyone who has fretted that their body is starting to fall apart, and it is for anyone who wants to prevent that happening in the future. It is a programme that will work 100 per cent of the time.

If you have posture-related issues and a sedentary lifestyle, when you make that first step and go to the gym, you can end up compounding the problems. You're taking a posture damaged by sitting down for too long during the day into a gym and loading it with weights or running with it. You are compounding an already dysfunctional operating system. You might do your gym programme for 4–6 weeks and then perhaps you'll get injured and so you'll say, 'That's it – I tried to get fit and look what happened.' People get trapped in a negative cycle – they start a new regime too quickly and end up quitting it entirely.

It's like building a Lego tower on bricks that have been incorrectly laid from the start. You'll keep adding more and more bricks until eventually it will topple over. What you actually need is to get back to basics and reset the fundamentals: your posture, your way of moving, your way of being.

This holds true when starting a programme like mine. To make a long-term, positive change you will have to analyse and inevitably change the way you act. To correct your physical imbalances and postural habits, you will have to implement conscious movement into your daily life. Doing my 21-minute workout each day reinforces your new movement patterns. I'm not offering a short-term solution, though. There is no magic, instant fix. You have to look at this as a long-term undertaking – a life transformation.

The first 21 days of the movement programme is the Body Reset Programme and is the same for everybody. Whether you have a knee problem, a back problem, a shoulder problem or a neck problem, you will have a movement problem.

The medical world likes to segment the body into different parts because it is easier to manage that way, but the body doesn't really work like that. If you injure your back, the medical community will usually isolate your back saying, 'This is the part that hurts, let's focus on that.' That often translates as, 'Let's inject your back!' But the problem is not your back. It's your body. And the root cause of why your back hurts is a movement problem.

Whatever part of your body is injured, you have to think about it in an integrated way in order to fix it. You don't fix your back; you fix yourself. You don't fix the part; you fix the whole. This is why you have to see a joined-up picture to be a good personal trainer – the whole jigsaw puzzle, not just one piece.

There will be parts of the exercise programme that are easy for you but your friend will find really difficult, and parts that you will find tough and your friend will breeze through. You need to stick at the hard stuff and not skip the easy stuff – it is all important.

This programme will put you under a significant amount of stress. There will be peaks and troughs in your fitness journey.

To help with the post-exercise aches and to avoid injuries, I will also teach you how to use my self-care Body Dynamix muscle massage programme (in the Forever Fix section on page 228). It will show you how to recognise problems that are creeping up on you and help you fix them.

FIRST STEPS

Aim to walk 10,000 steps per day. You can count this using your phone or a pedometer. If you are already hitting that target, aim for 25% more than your current daily average.

On average, people take 100-130 steps per minute, so if you walked around while speaking on the phone, walked to the office from one bus stop earlier than you normally would plus a 20-minute walk at lunch, you will easily reach this target. As an extra bonus, not sitting down all that time will accelerate correcting your postural imbalances by reinforcing your new conscious way of moving.

7 ASSESSMENT TESTS

IN MY EXPERIENCE, 90 PER CENT OF PEOPLE STRUGGLE WITH:

• Forward-leading head and rounded shoulders leading to neck and upper back pain.
• Weak lower back and inactive glutes.
• Lack of core awareness and hip inflexibility.

When you start this programme, you are likely to feel disconnected from your body. But as you move through it, you will learn how to spot your problem areas, learn how to fix these issues and end up with better posture and a balanced body.

Before you start my programme, we need to find out where you are at. So first follow my 7 assessment tests. I suggest you video yourself, so you can see how your body moves and spot improvements later.

THE 21-DAY BODY RESET PROGRAMME WILL:

• Activate your glutes (the muscles in your bottom), and correct lower back and pelvic movement.
• Improve hip flexibility.
• Strengthen your core and integrate movement with your hips and pelvis.

Repeat these tests in week 10 and then in week 16 – you should notice a big difference in your score.

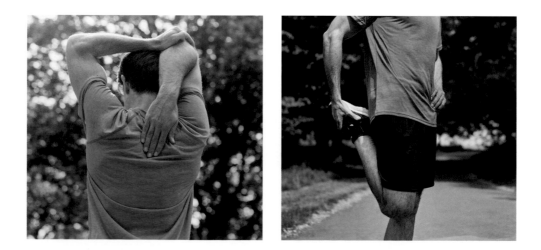

RESULTS

Add up the number of points to give yourself a final score. It's not a pass or a fail test – it's more about being able to see improvement when you repeat these exercises in weeks 10 and 16. However, it is a good guide of where you are to begin with. This is just an indication of where you are at now, to help you recognise where you need to improve and also where you are aiming to get to.

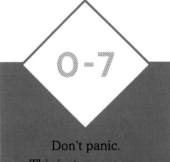

0-7

Don't panic.
This just means you
have work to do – the
21-day Body Reset
Programme will show
you how to improve.

7-14

Not bad, but we want
you scoring even
better.

14-21

Well done! But even if
you have scored highly,
there is always room for
improvement. You should
be aiming for full marks
by the end of the
16-week programme.

Test 1

UPPER BACK FLEXIBILITY

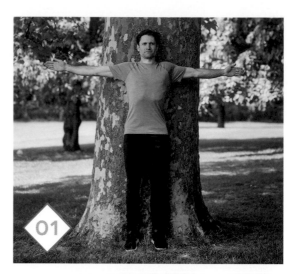

This test is to see how your head, shoulders and upper back are working together.

01. Find a flat wall (or tree) and stand against it. Place your back up against the wall, with your heels, buttocks, shoulders and head all touching it. Extend your arms out horizontally in a crucifix position.

02. Bend your elbows at 90 degrees, placing the backs of your hands on the wall with your palms facing forward and your fingertips pointing up to the sky. Engage your core (you should feel your abdomen tighten), adjusting the pelvis (your trunk between your stomach and thighs) and rib cage into a neutral position (see page 33). You do not want to be excessively arching through your lower back.

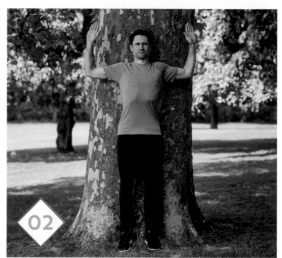

03. Slide your arms slowly up the wall and back down again.

DO YOU HAVE:

Normal mobility – able to move your upper arms close to your ears, without pain or restriction of movement (3 points)
Some pain / restriction in movement (2 points)
Restricted or very painful movement – unable to raise your arms completely, with some upper / mid back tightness (1 point)
Unable to raise your arms at all (0)

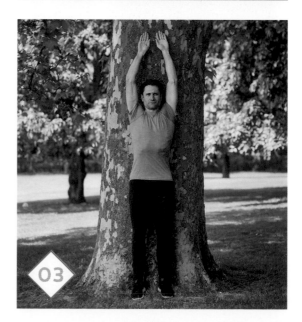

Test 2

HIP HINGE

This tests the mobility in (surprise!) your hips. Sitting down for long periods can make you forget how to hinge at your hips and how to use your glutes (the muscles in your bottom).

01. Stand with your feet hip width apart.

02. Lock yourself into a neutral position (see image on page 33) through the hips with straight legs and a flat, straight back.

03. Hinge forward at the hips. You should be able to reach 90 degrees without rounding your shoulders or spine.

DO YOU FIND THIS:

Easy (3 points)
Somewhat difficult (2 points)
Difficult – you have some pain (1 point)
Impossible – you cannot reach 90 degrees or your shoulders round. You need to have a flat, straight back (0)

NOTE:
Use a pole, mop or broom handle to help guide the movement. Rest the pole along your back and hold it above your head and at the base of your spine to stop you rounding your back as you hinge.

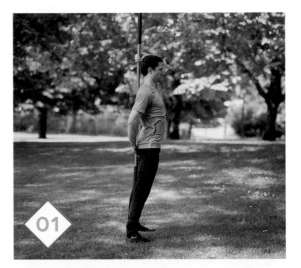

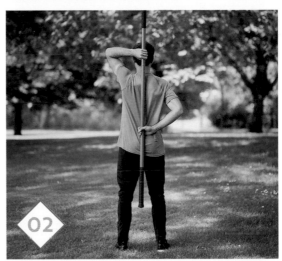

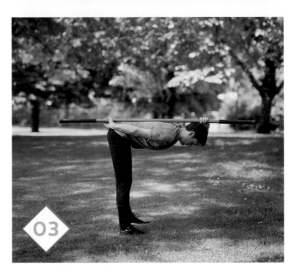

Test 3

STANDING SQUAT

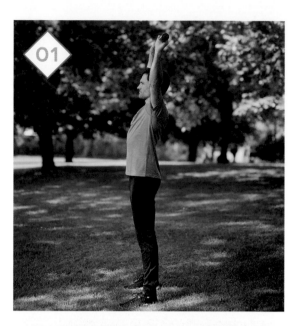

If you can't keep your arms above your head throughout the movement, you need to work on your upper back, shoulder flexibility and core strength. If you can't squat down the whole way, you need to work on your calf, hamstring and hip flexibility and on the strength of your glutes.

01. Stand with your feet hip width apart and your arms extended up to the ceiling.

02. Bend your knees and keep your back straight as you drop down into a squat.

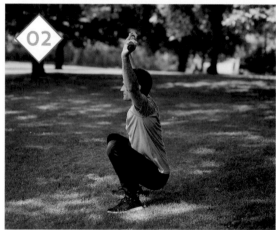

03. Return to a standing position.

DO YOU FIND THIS:

Easy (3 points)
Somewhat difficult (2 points)
Difficult (1 point)
Impossible (0)

If you round your shoulders or can't get down to a 45-degree knee bend, or if you are unable to return to a standing position, you score 0.

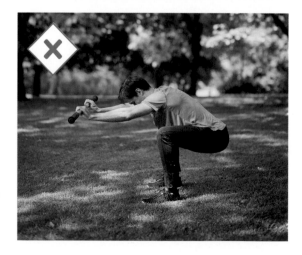

NOTE:

Put a rolled-up small towel under both heels and perform the squat again. Does that help? If so, you are most likely to be suffering from tight hips, tight hamstrings and/or tight calf muscles.

Test 4

GLUTE STRENGTH

If your knee buckles inward, it shows that the muscles in your bottom and your feet aren't strong enough.

01. Stand with your feet hip width apart. Lift your left leg in front of you and hold it elevated off the floor.

02. Standing on your right leg, perform a single leg squat.

03. Repeat on the other leg.

DO YOU FIND THIS:

Easy (3 points)
Somewhat difficult (2 points)
Difficult (1 point)
Impossible (0)

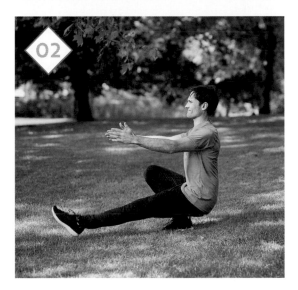

Can you squat and stand back up again without your knee collapsing inward? If your knee collapses, it is most likely because your glutes (the muscles in your bottom) are not working as they should to support your body throughout the movement. You score 0 if you can't deep squat and stand back up again without your knee collapsing inward.

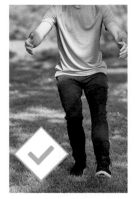
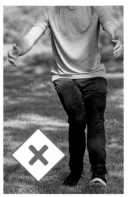

49

Test 5

ROTATION

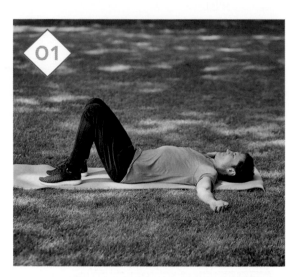

This tests spinal and shoulder mobility. If you can't lower your knees to the ground comfortably while keeping both shoulders on the ground, then you have work to do.

01. Lie down on your back on the floor with your arms out to the side and your knees bent.

02. Slowly lower your knees to the left side, maintaining the 90-degree bend, and simultaneously turn your head to the opposite side, without lifting your head or shoulders off the ground.

Return to the starting position.

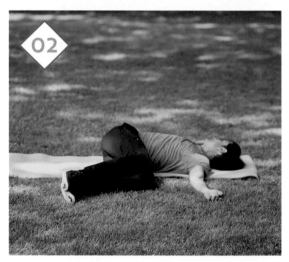

03. Repeat on the other side.

DO YOU FIND THIS:
Easy (3 points)
Somewhat difficult (2 points)
Difficult (1 point)
Impossible (0)

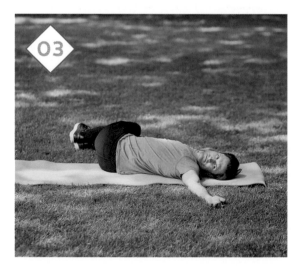

Test 6

CORE ENGAGEMENT

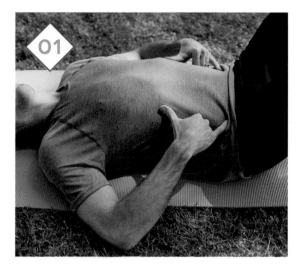

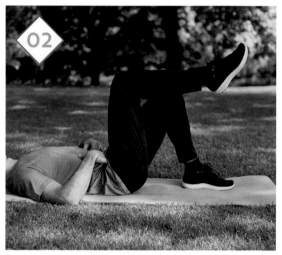

This tests the engagement of your core muscles – the muscles around your trunk.

01. Lie on your back with your knees bent and your feet flat on the ground. Place your hands across your stomach, resting your thumbs on your last rib and your little fingers touching your pelvic crests (the top of your hip bones). Pull your ribs down slightly and tilt your pelvis so that your pelvic crest bones move towards the rib cage (where your thumbs are resting).

02. Maintaining this position, tighten your stomach muscles. In order to understand how to do this, cough and hold that abdominal tension in your core. Now, release it a little so that you can still breathe. Holding this conscious core engagement (in other words your stomach muscles are 'on'), breathe out slightly as you raise your right foot, maintaining the 90-degree

bend in the knee. Take a shallow breath in, then exhale as you raise the left leg up to meet the right. Breathe in at the top and out as you lower your right leg.

03. Alternate and repeat until you've done 20 reps.

DO YOU FIND THIS:

Easy (3 points)
Somewhat difficult (2 points)
Difficult (1 point)
Impossible (0)

NOTE:
Learning to integrate breathing with engaged stomach muscles is the same feeling as when you're trying to blow up a strong balloon. You have to keep the tension and breathe simultaneously.

Test 7

PELVIC TILT

This test will help you understand how your hips are currently moving. You need to perform the same movement in 3 different positions: lying flat; on all fours; and standing.

This test is graded differently: 1 point for a pass or 0 if you're unable to do it.

NOTE:
It will help if you do this in front of a mirror. Many people find their chin pitches forward or their shoulders round, hunching the upper back.

LYING FLAT

ANTERIOR PELVIC TILT

01. Lie on your back on the floor with your knees bent and feet flat on the ground.

02. Tilt your hips, arching your lower back off the floor, creating a tunnel underneath your spine. Keep your feet, hips, head and shoulders resting on the floor.

POSTERIOR PELVIC TILT

03. This is the opposite of the above. Lie on your back on the floor with your knees bent and feet flat on the ground.

04. Flatten your back on to the floor, so that there is no gap between your back and the floor. Keep your feet, hips, head and shoulders resting on the floor.

If you can do these 2 movements, you get 1 point. If you can't, you get 0.

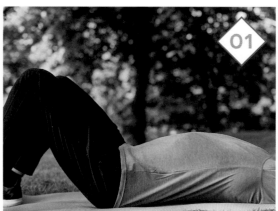

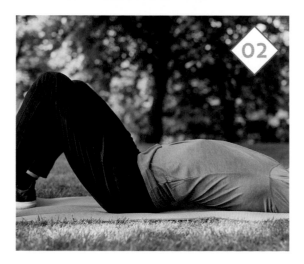

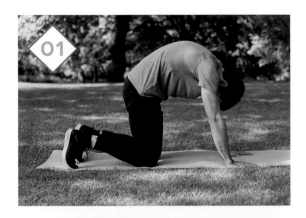

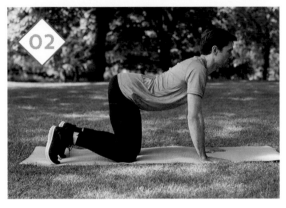

ON ALL FOURS

01. Get on your hands and knees. Taking a deep breath in, arch your spine up to the ceiling (the 'cow stretch').

02. Now perform the opposite (the 'cat stretch'), lowering your hips and arching your back, sinking your spine to the floor to create a large dip between your head and hips.

If you can do these 2 movements, you get 1 point. If you can't, you get 0.

STANDING

01. With your hands on your hips, tuck your hips underneath you. Imagine you have a tail and you are tucking it between your legs.

02. Now, do the opposite. Arch your lower back, tilting your spine to create an accentuated lower back curve. You must make sure nothing else (such as your head, neck or shoulders) is moving.

03. Try not to round your shoulders or pitch your head forward as you do it.

If you can do this pelvic tilt without any other body parts moving, you get 1 point. If you can't, you get 0.

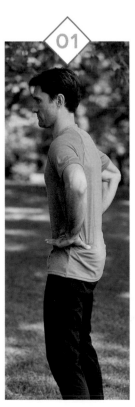

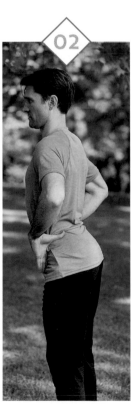

53

THE PROGRAMME IN FULL

WEEKS 1–3

EXERCISE:
Body Reset Programme (see pages 56–95) every day for 21 minutes.

FOOD:
1 day a week eating only 500 calories; 1 day a week off; every other day eating in an 8-hour window (making sure you are not eating for 16 hours).

WEEKS 4–9

EXERCISE:
Transformational Programme (see pages 102–127) 5 days out of 7 each week for 21 minutes. You are integrating what you have learned about exercise into a more dynamic workout.

FOOD:
4 days a week eating within an 8-hour window (making sure you are not eating for 16 hours); 3 days a week eating at any time.

If you fall off the wagon, go back to the Body Reset Programme.

WEEK 10

EXERCISE:
Return to the Body Reset Programme week 3 (see pages 82–95) every day for 21 minutes.

FOOD:
1 day a week eating only 500 calories; 1 day a week off; every other day eating in an 8-hour window (making sure you are not eating for 16 hours).

WEEKS 11–16

EXERCISE:
Return to the Transformational Programme (see pages 102–127) 5 days out of 7 each week for 21 minutes.

FOOD:
4 days a week eating within an 8-hour window (making sure you are not eating for 16 hours); 3 days a week eating at any time.

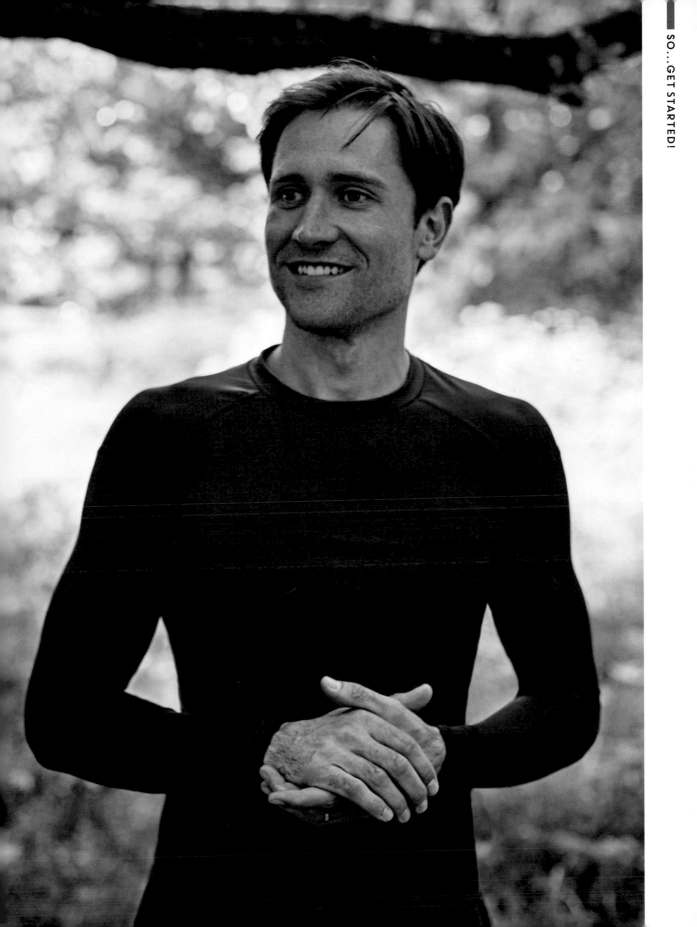

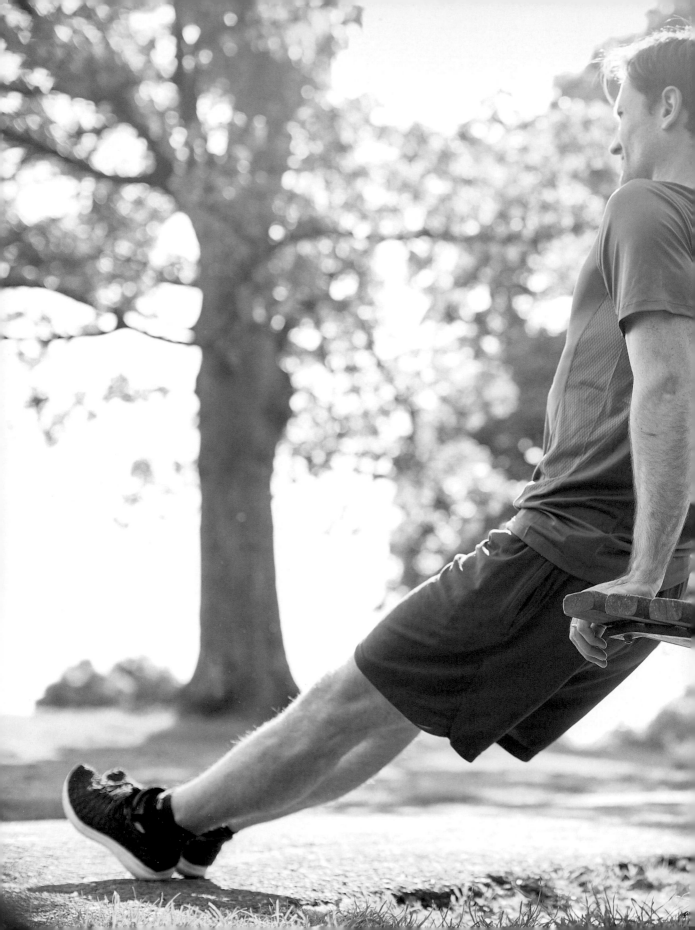

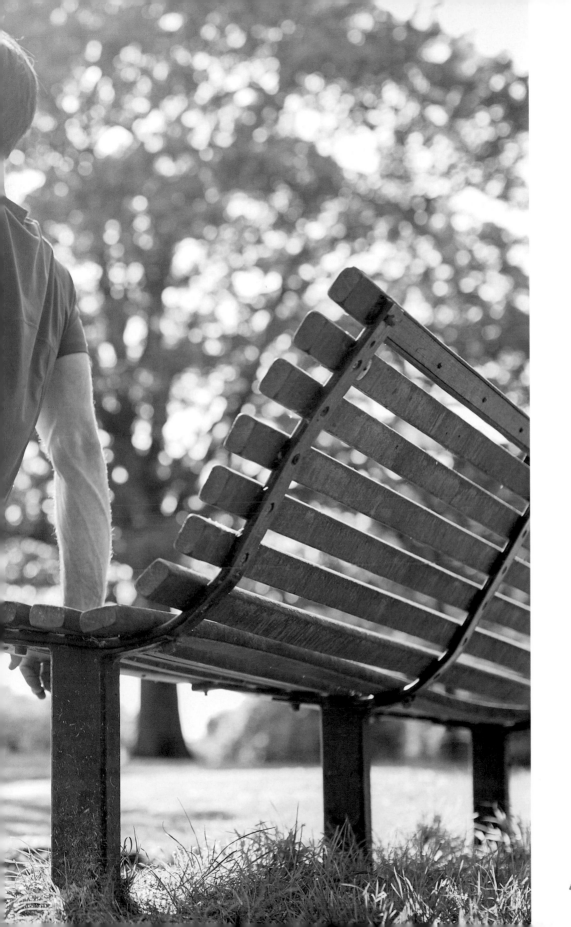

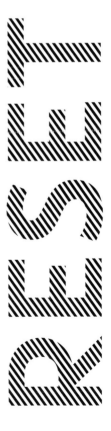

PART ONE

RESET

/21 DAYS

WORKOUTS

In technical terms, what we're doing is 'deconstructing your movement into its foundational pieces'. We're going to teach the body the different types of movement – extension, rotation and flexion. There are parts of the body that need mobilising and other parts that need strengthening. Once you've completed the reset phase, you will integrate the two.

On paper, the exercise part of the 3-week programme may look easy. It's just 21 minutes a day for 21 days. But these 21 days are about changing the way you move and about fixing your body – getting you ready for the next part of the programme. I want your new way of moving to be drilled into your mind by the time the 21 days are up.

Once you have finished the reset, you can start the Transformational Programme, a more physically exhausting set of exercises. Continue doing this programme until week 10, when you should return to a week of Reset. Finally, in weeks 11–16 you will go back to the Transformational Programme.

WALKING TEST

Before you start you need to take a walking-on-the-spot test. It's simple and . . . amusing.

- Find a space where you have some room to move around.
- Set up a camera to record your movements or get a friend to help you.
- Set up a timer and time for 2 minutes.
- Close your eyes or put on a blindfold (no peeking and cheating!).
- March on the spot, swinging your arms and raising your knees. Sing your favourite song as you march.
- When the timer goes, open your eyes and see where you are now standing.

If you are in the same place as when you started, well done! I've never seen anyone manage it. For everyone else, this exercise is designed to show you that you're off balance. There could be a pelvic twist or you could be leading from the right side of your body, perhaps you're rotating as you march or your centre of gravity is slightly behind your centre. Whatever your individual result, it shows that your body is moving with imbalances.

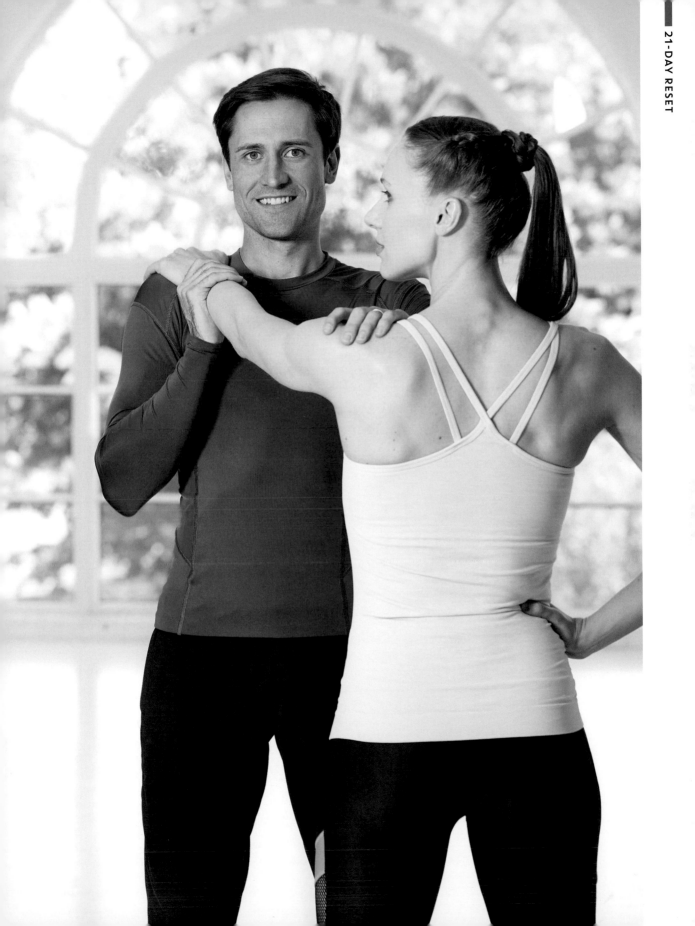

Week 1.

(Do these exercises every day for 7 days.)

Week 1 focuses on building the foundations of core and glute strength and mobility. Consciously focusing on these exercises is the cornerstone to correcting your posture. Don't worry if it hurts. Remember: the more you do it, the more your body will adapt. You are now on the path to a pain-free life. The exercise routine may take more than 21 minutes when you're starting out. As you improve you'll become faster.

• **Most of the exercises flow into the next seamlessly.**
• **You will need a towel and an exercise mat.**
• **Do the exercises barefoot.**

FOR ALL OF THESE EXERCISES...

There are 3 Golden Rules, whether you are standing, lying or on all fours:

01. You need to set your head, neck and shoulders - tuck your chin in slightly to your neck, as you would if you're trying to look down your nose, and pull your shoulders back and down.

02. Pull down your rib cage, brace your core and tilt your hips so you're holding a neutral spine (see image above and page 33).

03. Grip the floor with your toes to maintain a natural foot arch and glute activation.

NOW YOU ARE READY FOR THE EXERCISES.

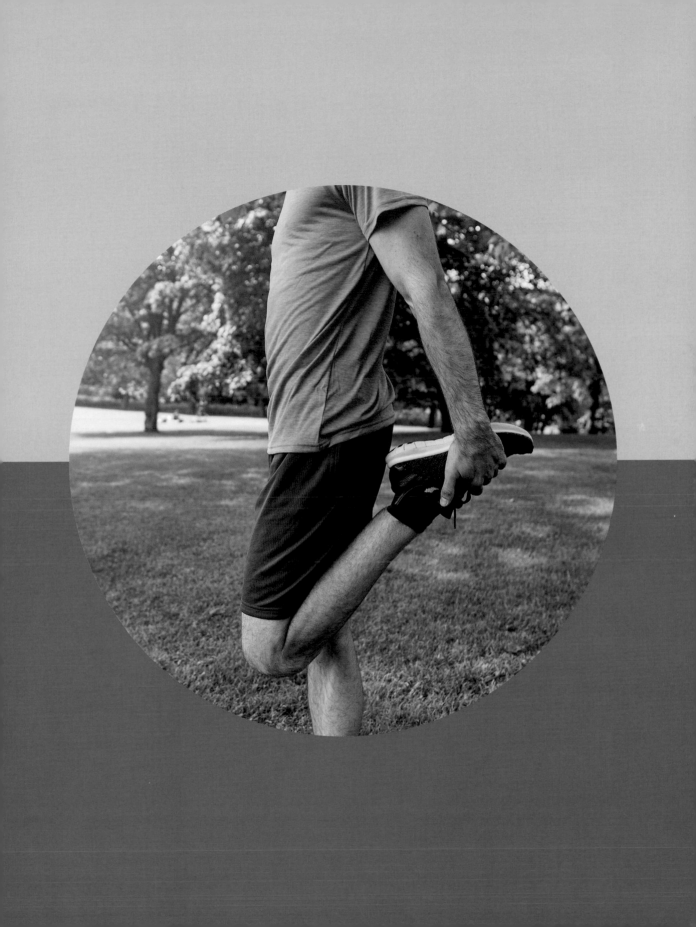

LEG LIFTS

01. Start on all fours with your hands directly below your shoulders and your knees below your hips. Pull your shoulders back and down to get tension under your armpits. Make sure the creases in your elbows are pointing forward. Pull your hips and rib cage closer than feels normal. That will keep you stable.

02. Once you have the starting position correct, stretch your left leg out straight behind you. Apply a little pressure on to the back foot – rock back slightly.

03. Slowly lower and lift that foot 20 times. Make sure you are squeezing your left butt cheek as you do it.

04. Return to all fours.

05. Reset to the start position with your back and neck straight, your elbow creases forward and your ribs and hips engaged.

06. Repeat the exercise with your right leg. Make sure your butt cheek is performing the lift.

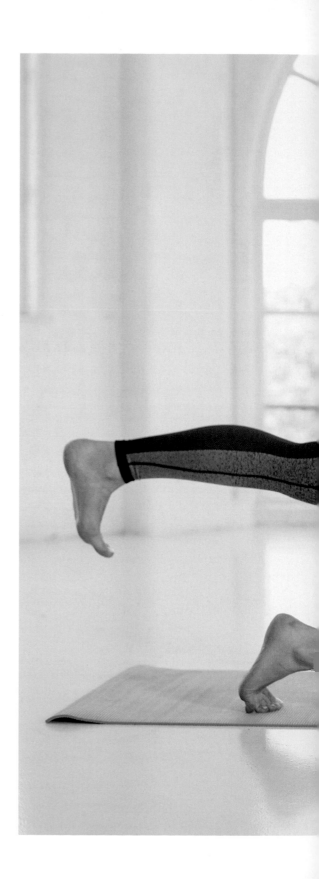

You want a natural arch in your back - try to maintain tension in your stomach.

Make sure you don't drop your head. Imagine there's a door lying across your back so your back, neck and head make a straight line.

THE
PIGEON

01. Starting on all fours, straighten your right leg behind you, with your toes resting on the floor.

02. Bring your left leg forward in front of you, crossing it underneath your body so much of your weight is resting on the left leg. You should feel this in your left butt cheek.

03. Sink down, with your elbows bent underneath your shoulders. Rock from side to side.

04. Hold the stretch for 30 seconds.

05. Switch positions and repeat with your left leg straightened and your right leg forward.

The calf of your left leg should be at 90 degrees to your right leg. You should feel this in your left butt cheek. Make sure you remain slightly elevated – don't sit down!

CHILD'S POSE

01. Starting on all fours, rest your bottom on the heels of your feet, with your arms reaching forward and your toes pointed behind you.

02. Drop your head and breathe.

03. Hold for 30 seconds.

If your arms feel too tight, you can bend your elbows.

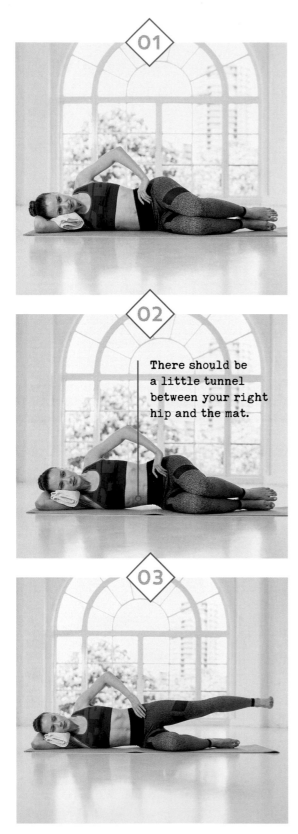

There should be a little tunnel between your right hip and the mat.

LYING LEG CIRCLES

01. Lie on your right side with your knees bent. Fold up a towel and rest your head on it. Bend your arm under the towel as well – or extend your arm out if that's more comfortable.

02. Focusing on your hips and rib cage, lift your rib cage off the floor and push your hips away from you, towards your feet. Roll slightly forward.

03. Extend your left leg out, keeping the tunnel underneath you. Move your left leg backward and forward. Make sure you are squeezing your left butt cheek as you do it.

04. Repeat 20 times.

05. Circle your leg slowly clockwise 20 times. Your squeezed butt cheek should be performing the movement.

06. Now reverse: circle your leg slowly anti-clockwise 20 times.

07. Change sides and repeat the exercises.

GLUTE STRETCH

01. Lie down on your back with your knees bent and your feet flat on the floor.

02. Cross your right ankle over your left knee.

03. Bring your left leg up to a 90-degree angle and interlink your fingers behind the thigh of your left leg. Hold for 20 seconds.

04. Relax your position then change sides and repeat the exercises.

05. Hug your knees to your chest for 10 seconds.

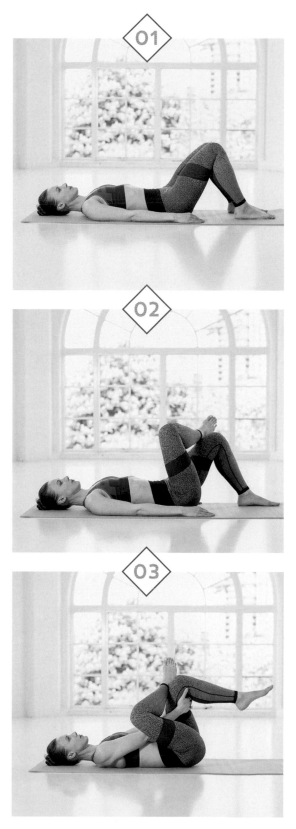

67

Imagine that you have a tattoo numbering 1-5 running down your lower back - put each number down in turn, with 1 (on your bottom) being the last to touch the ground.

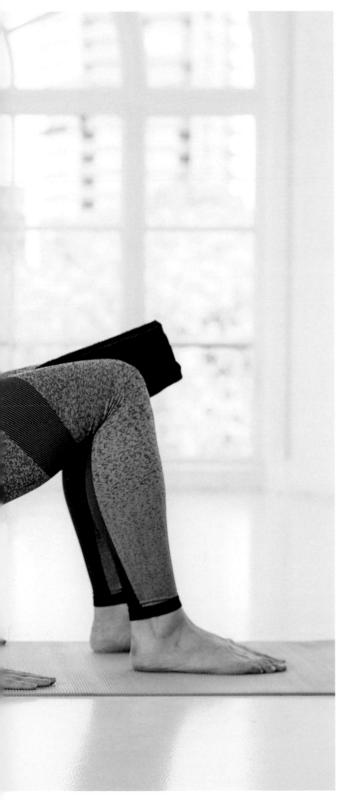

BACK FIXER BRIDGE

01. Lie on your back with your knees bent and your feet flat on the floor.

02. Place a towel between your knees and bring your feet a foot's length away from your bottom. Squeeze the towel.

03. Roll your body up, lifting your bottom and lower back off the ground.

04. Slowly roll back down, placing your back down in sections.

05. Slowly roll your body back up in the same way, and then slowly roll back down again.

06. Repeat another 8 times.

CORE ACTIVATION & ROTATION

01. Lie on your back with your knees bent and your feet flat on the floor.

02. Raise your right leg, so your knee is at a 90-degree bend.

03. Raise your left leg, so your knee is at a 90-degree bend, too.

04. Lower your right foot so your right heel touches the floor and lift it back up again.

05. Then lower your left foot and lift it back up again.

06. Repeat this 20 times on each side.

07. Hug your knees into your chest.

08. Place a towel between your knees and bring both legs up into a 90-degree bend, with your arms out to the side, making a crucifix position.

09. Roll your legs to the right as you look to the left (see page 50).

10. Roll your legs to the left as you look to the right.

11. Repeat 20 times on each side.

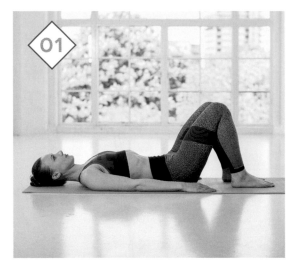

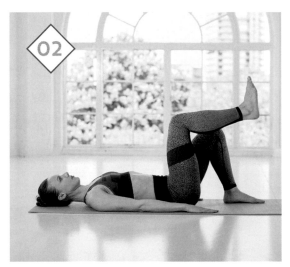

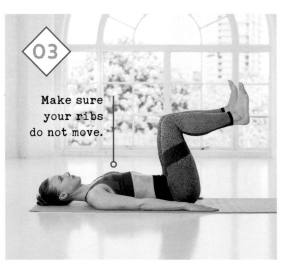

Make sure your ribs do not move.

HIP FLEXOR STRETCH

01. Position yourself with your left knee kneeling down and your right foot forward flat on the mat. Squeeze your right butt cheek.

With your arms out in front of you, reach forward with your upper body. Hold for 5 seconds then move your upper body back again. Repeat 10 times.

Swap your legs over and repeat 10 times.

02. Swap back to kneeling on your left knee and do the same movement, but with your arms reaching up towards the ceiling. Repeat 10 times.

Swap your legs over and repeat 10 times.

Switch back to kneeling on the left leg and do the same movement reaching upwards but include a side bend from the hip after you have reached up with your arms. Repeat 10 times.

Swap your legs over and repeat 10 times.

03. Switch back to kneeling on the left knee and reach forward, then rotate your upper body to the left, opening out your arms. Move your body back to the centre. Repeat 10 times.

Swap your legs over and repeat 10 times.

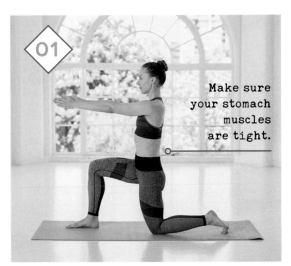

Make sure your stomach muscles are tight.

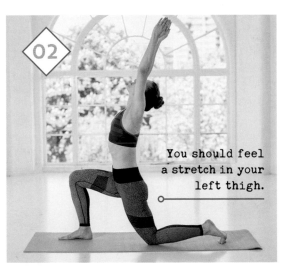

You should feel a stretch in your left thigh.

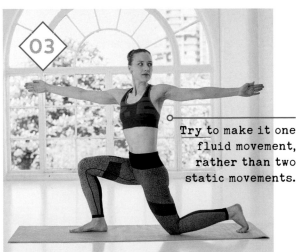

Try to make it one fluid movement, rather than two static movements.

71

Week 2.

(Do these exercises every day for 7 days.)

Using a foam roller introduces you to places in your body that have trigger points (or muscle tightness). Releasing this build-up of muscle tension from years of moving inefficiently will help correct your poor movement patterns. By releasing overworked muscles, you encourage smaller postural muscles to do their job. This may hurt a little – but it's 'good pain'.

- **You will need a foam roller, as well as a towel and an exercise mat. You can buy foam rollers from sports shops, department stores or online.**
- **Do the exercises barefoot.**

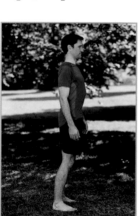

FOR ALL OF THESE EXERCISES...

There are 3 Golden Rules, whether you are standing, lying or on all fours:

01. You need to set your head, neck and shoulders - tuck your chin in slightly to your neck, as you would if you're trying to look down your nose, and pull your shoulders back and down.

02. Pull down your rib cage, brace your core and tilt your hips so you're holding a neutral spine (see image above and page 33).

03. Grip the floor with your toes to maintain a natural foot arch and glute activation.

NOW YOU ARE READY FOR THE EXERCISES.

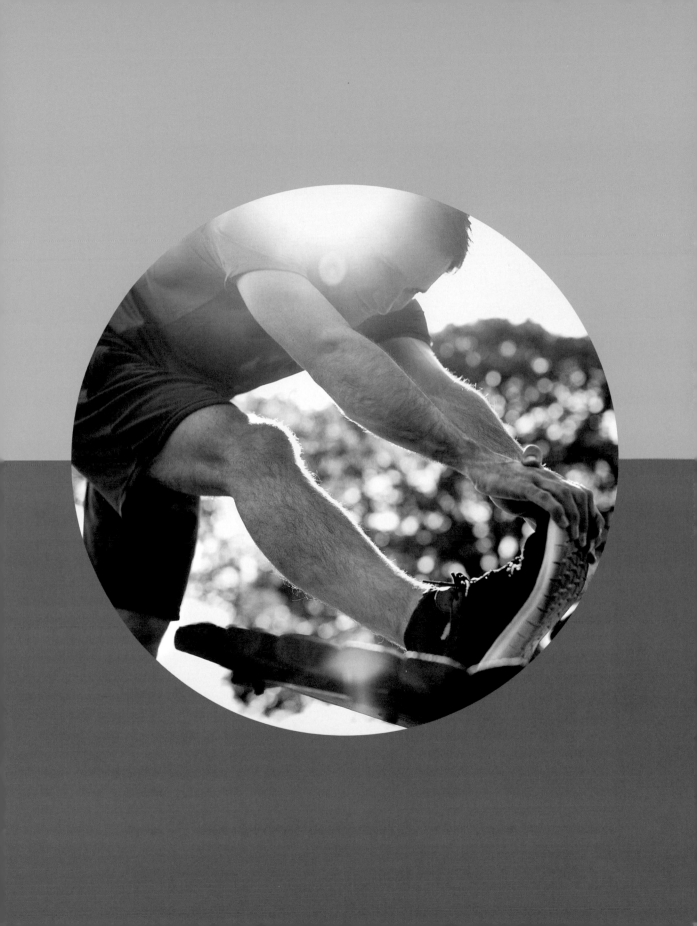

LOVE YOUR BUNS

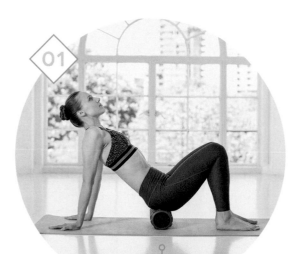

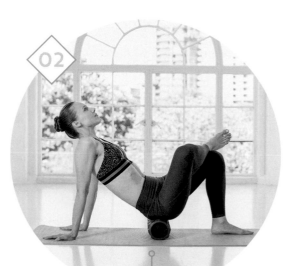

Make sure
you are
relaxing your
muscle tension.

You don't need to
move the roller
far - just a few
inches.

01. Sit down with the foam roller under your bottom, your knees bent and arms behind you, hands facing away.

02. Place your right ankle on your left knee and begin rolling. Everyone rolls the muscle 'north to south' but don't forget to roll 'east to west' if you find a sore spot. Make sure you are relaxing your muscle tension.

03. When you start to feel comfortable, move around and find another sore spot.

HIP FLEXORS

01. Rest on your right side with the foam roller beneath you. Use your right arm to prop yourself up and place your left arm in front of you. Bring your left leg over your right leg. Roll yourself forward slightly, using your arms to propel your body forward, so that the roller is resting right at the top of your thigh.

02. Now bring yourself further up, so that the roller is under the middle of your right thigh. Turn on to your front. Your right thigh should be on the roller with your arms bent in front of you and your left leg should be bent out to the side in a resting position.

03. Once you have found a sore spot on the front of your thigh, bend your right knee. Straighten your leg out once again and continue rolling toward the knee. Repeat every time you come across a tender area. Continue rolling until you are just above your knee.

04. Reset to the start position then turn on to your left side on the roller and repeat the exercises.

It took me a good few weeks to do this without tears in my eyes!

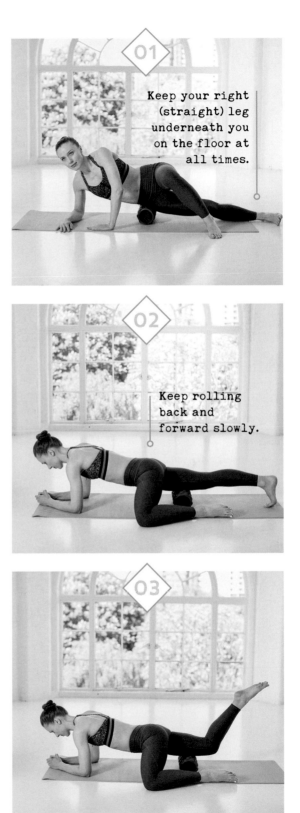

Keep your right (straight) leg underneath you on the floor at all times.

Keep rolling back and forward slowly.

LYING LEG CIRCLES

01. Lie on your left side with your knees bent. Extend your left arm up under your head and place a towel between your head and your arm.

02. Focus on your hips and rib cage. Lift your rib cage off the floor and push your hips away from you, towards your feet. Roll slightly forward. Extend the right leg, keeping the tunnel underneath your hip.

03. Squeezing your right butt cheek, move your right leg backward and forward.

04. Repeat 25 times, making sure the hip doesn't collapse into the mat.

05. Now circle your leg slowly clockwise 25 times. Your squeezed butt cheek should be performing the movement.

06. Reverse the direction and circle your leg slowly anti-clockwise. Repeat 25 times.

07. Change sides and repeat the exercises.

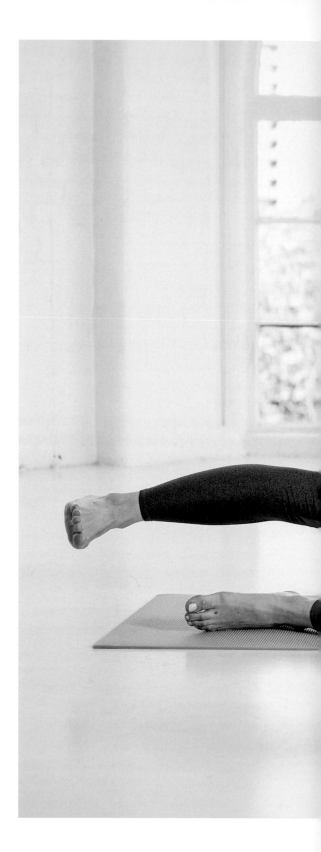

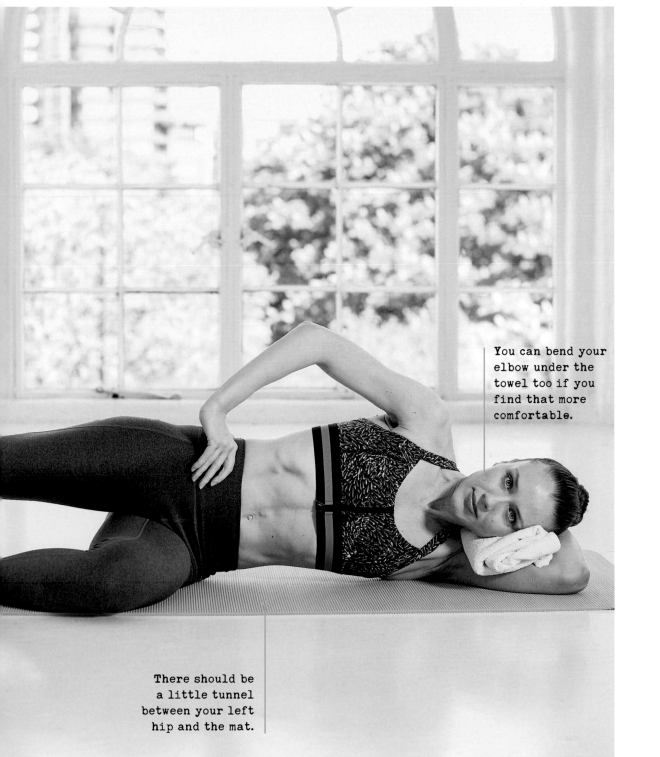

You can bend your
elbow under the
towel too if you
find that more
comfortable.

There should be
a little tunnel
between your left
hip and the mat.

LEG STRETCH

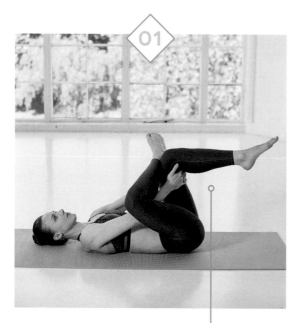

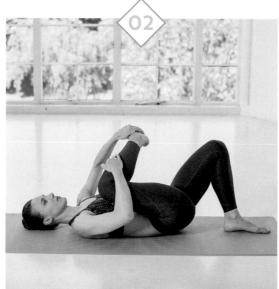

Interlink your hands behind your left thigh and pull your leg in.

01. Lie on your back with your knees bent. Cross your right leg over your left, placing your right ankle on your left knee. Interlink your hands behind your left thigh and pull your leg in.

02. If you are already very flexible, you can let go of your left thigh and take hold of your bent right leg, pulling it into the body, with your right knee towards your right shoulder. Gently hug your leg so the right knee is close to your right shoulder.

03. Repeat with the other leg.

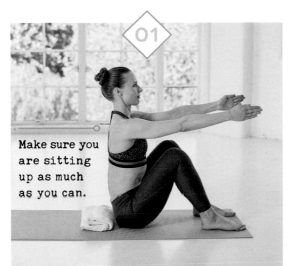

01

Make sure you are sitting up as much as you can.

ROLL BACKS

01. Sit with your knees bent with the towel rolled up behind your bottom, if you need it. Extend your arms out in front of you.

02. Roll backward slowly using your hips, only reaching your arms over your head once you are lying down.

03. Come back up into a sitting position – raising your arms first, then tightening the stomach to sit up.

04. Repeat 15 times – really focus on doing it properly each time.

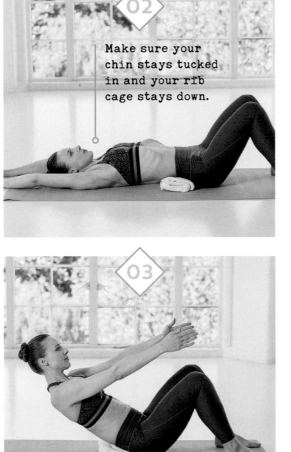

02

Make sure your chin stays tucked in and your rib cage stays down.

03

CAT STRETCH

Your eyes should be looking straight ahead.

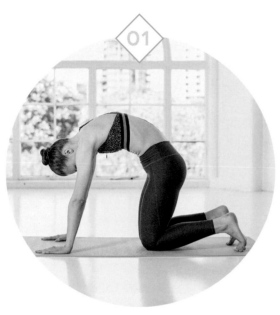

01. Starting on all fours, arch your back, pushing your chest to the ceiling. Your head should drop down towards the floor.

02. Now sink your chest down to the floor – dropping the shoulders. Make sure you are doing this slowly.

03. Repeat 15 times – each time trying to reach a bit further.

04. Finally, sit back on your heels and reach your arms out in front of you. Lower your forehead down on to the mat into Child's Pose (see page 65).

SNAKE

01. Lie down on your front and rest your forehead on a towel. Your chin should be tucked in and your arms at your sides. Inhale.

02. Keeping the tension in your ribs and hips, exhale as you squeeze your glutes and arch your back, which will lift your head about 3cm off the towel. As your head, chest and shoulders lift up, so do your arms and hands as one unit. Feel as though you are reaching your thumbs up to the ceiling as you extend off the mat. This will help maintain a retracted shoulder blade position.

03. Inhale at the top of the movement and hold for 1 second, then exhale as you lower back down slowly.

04. Repeat 15 times.

Make sure you are not lifting your chin and looking in front of you.

Make sure your ribs and hips are connected and crunched - they should be 'on'.

Week 3.

(Do these exercises every day for 7 days.)

Week 3 will challenge you more on the roller. The Golden Rules should be ingrained now while you perform the exercises. That means you can focus on all three fundamental movements of the body – extension, rotation and flexion. Training your body to perform these movements correctly reduces the risk of muscle and joint pain, and will give you a strong, resilient body.

• **You will need a towel, an exercise mat, a foam roller, a mini loop band and a resistance loop band.**

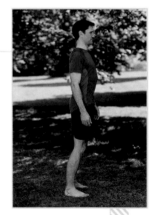

FOR ALL OF THESE EXERCISES...

There are 3 Golden Rules, whether you are standing, lying or on all fours:

01. You need to set your head, neck and shoulders - tuck your chin in slightly to your neck, as you would if you're trying to look down your nose, and pull your shoulders back and down.

02. Pull down your rib cage, brace your core and tilt your hips so you're holding a neutral spine (see image above and page 33).

03. Grip the floor with your toes to maintain a natural foot arch and glute activation.

NOW YOU ARE READY FOR THE EXERCISES.

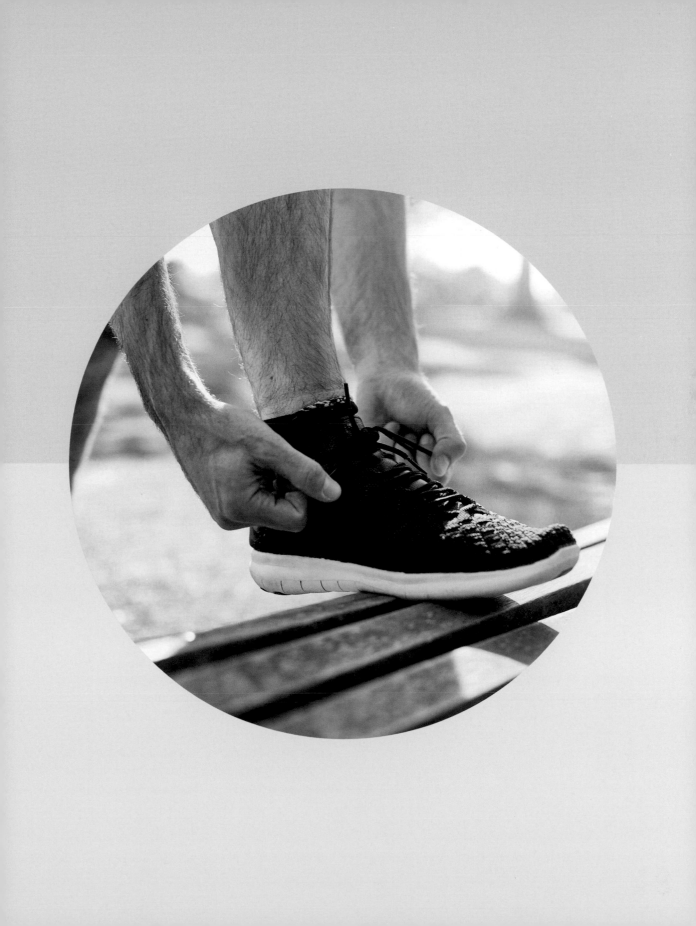

FOAM ROLLER CRUNCHES

Lean back
with your
hands behind
your head.

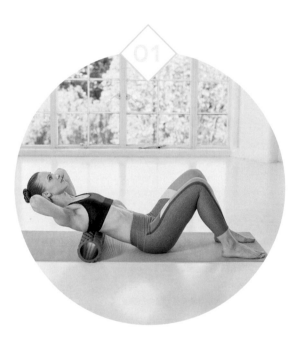

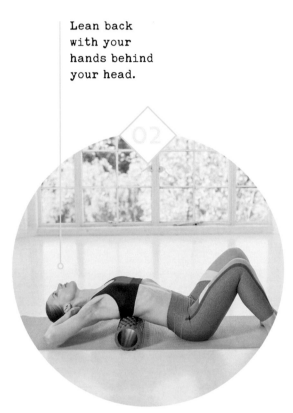

01. Lie on your back with the foam roller just below your shoulder blades. Bend your knees and place your feet flat on the floor.

02. Slowly lower your head back, arching yourself over the roller (remembering to take small, shallow breaths – do not hold your breath!). Only go as far as to make you feel a little discomfort – but make it a challenge. Crunch your abdominals (stomach muscles) to bring yourself back up. Reset and repeat 5 times.

You can adjust the foam roller with your hands to ensure it is in the best position.

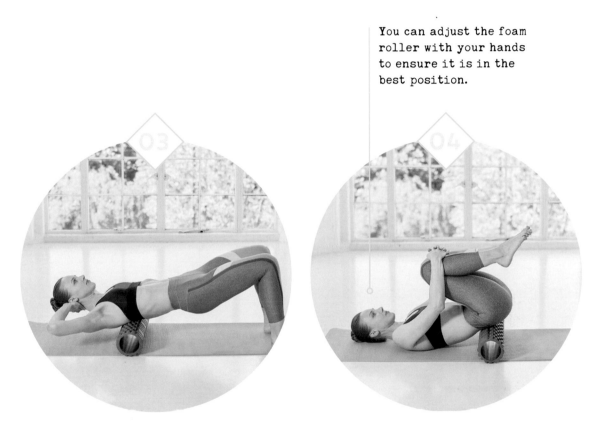

03. Lift your hips off the floor and roll down towards your hips a few centimetres. Lower your hips down to the floor again. Now repeat step 2. Continue to do this all the way down your spine until you reach your lower back.

04. When you get down to the base of your lower back, rest your head on the floor and tuck and tilt your hips over the roller. This is a small curved movement. Now rest for 20 seconds and hug your knees to your chest.

THE MILLION DOLLAR ROLL

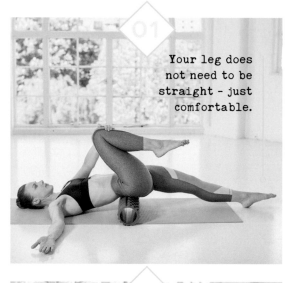

Your leg does not need to be straight - just comfortable.

01. Lie on your back and hug your knees to your chest. Position the roller comfortably under your hips and lower back. Release your left leg and rest your heel on the floor.

02. Twist your body anti-clockwise, bringing your right leg down to the left side as you look to the right. Hold that position for 10 seconds.

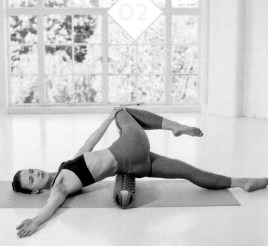

03. Rotate your upper back, bringing your right hand to your left, which should stay on the floor, clapping them together. Make sure you are breathing in when you come forward to clap your hands. Breathe out as you bring your right arm back to the right-hand side.

04. Repeat 20 times.

05. Reset to the start position then release your right leg and rest your heel on the floor. Repeat the exercises on the other side.

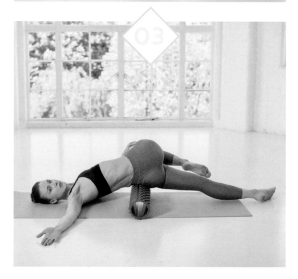

SHOULDER FIX

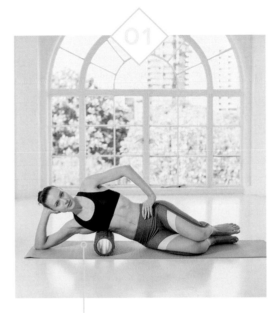

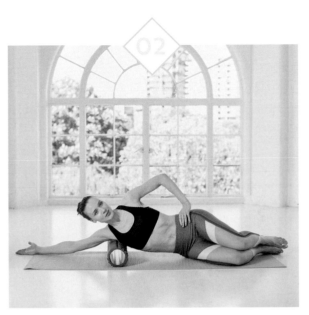

Rest your head in
your right hand
with your elbow
on the floor.

01. Lie on your right side and position the roller about half-way between your armpit and hip. Place your left hand on your left hip.

02. Slowly roll the roller up your body so that it travels towards your armpit, stopping whenever you find a sore spot.

03. Once you find a sore spot, move your right arm forward and back, with your palms facing up, as though you're mapping out a quarter of a circle.

04. Change sides and repeat the exercises.

87

HIP MOBILISER

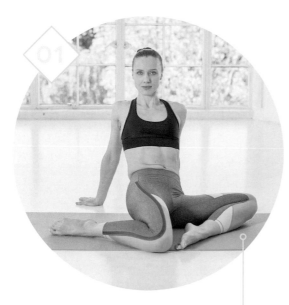

Don't worry if your knee can't quite touch the mat.

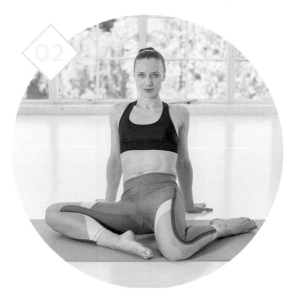

01. Sit up tall with both legs bent and flat on the floor. Your left leg should be positioned to create a triangle to your side with your left foot in front of you. Your right knee should be pointing forward and your right foot should be out to the side. Leave a small gap between your left heel and the upper part of your right leg.

02. Switch both legs from side to side 20 times. Make sure that your chest is facing forward, remaining fixed, and that all that moves are your hips and knees. If your bottom moves forward, shift it back to your starting position. The more you do this, the more comfortable the exercise will feel in your hips.

CLAMS

01. Lie on your right side and bend your right arm under your head. Place a towel between your arm and your head if that is more comfortable. Bend your knees at a 90-degree angle. Position a mini loop band around your thighs above your knee. Make sure there's a tunnel underneath your body and that your shoulder does not shrug. Rest your left hand on your left hip.

02. Lift your feet, so they are in line with the top of your hip.

03. Now lift and lower the top knee, making a kite shape with your legs. Breathe out as your knee lifts and squeeze your left butt cheek. That's the part of your body that should be doing the lifting. You can put your spare hand on your bum to make sure that muscle is working.

04. Repeat 20 times.

05. Change sides and repeat the exercises.

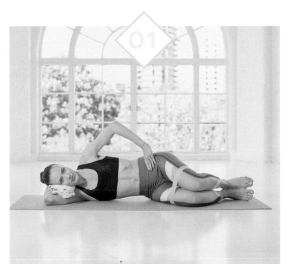

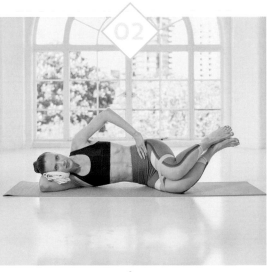

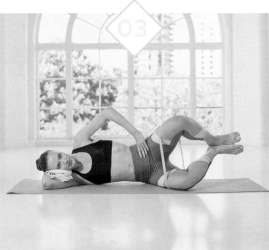

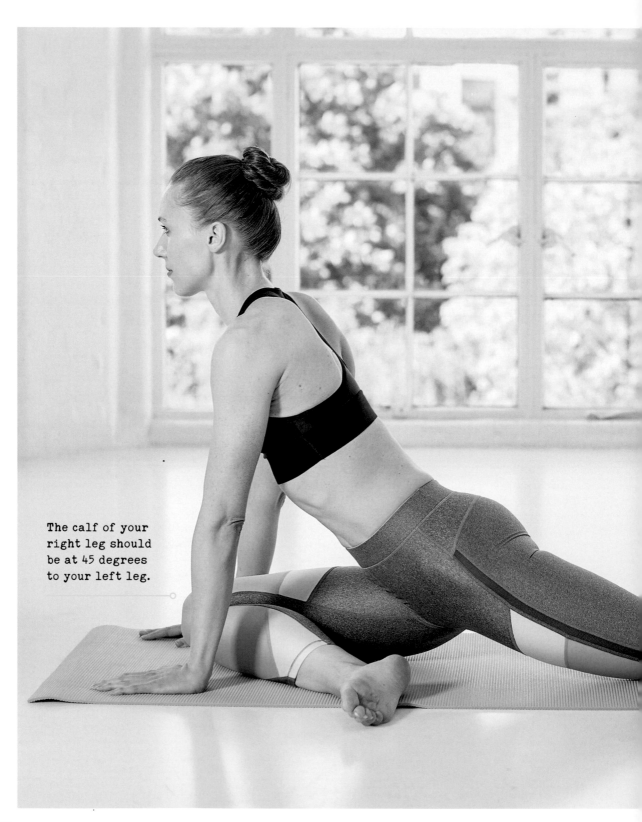

The calf of your right leg should be at 45 degrees to your left leg.

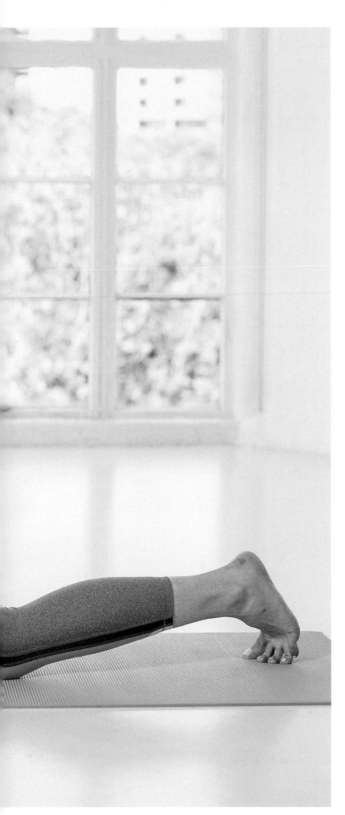

THE PIGEON

01. Starting on all fours, straighten your left leg behind you, with your toes resting on the floor.

02. Bring your right leg forward in front of you, crossing it underneath your body so much of your weight is resting on the right leg. You should feel this in your right butt cheek.

03. Sink down, with your elbows bent underneath your shoulders. Rock from side to side.

04. Hold the stretch for 30 seconds.

05. Switch positions and repeat with your right leg straightened and your left leg forward.

CHEST OPENING SALUTE

01. Start on all fours with your hands directly underneath your shoulders and your chin tucked in.

02. Put your left hand to your temple, as though you are giving a salute. (Do not put it on the back of your head, which will push your head down.)

03. Open your chest by raising your elbow and your eyes to the ceiling. Your chest, shoulder and head should move as you twist at the waist, but do not move your hips.

04. Repeat 20 times.

05. Reset to the start position then put your right hand to your temple and repeat the exercises on the other side.

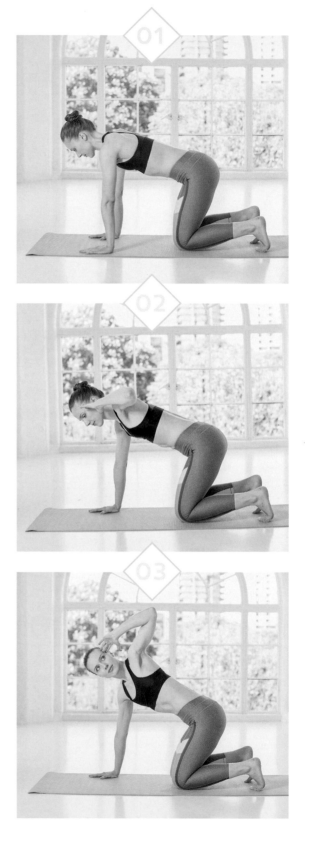

ALL FOURS LEG RAISES

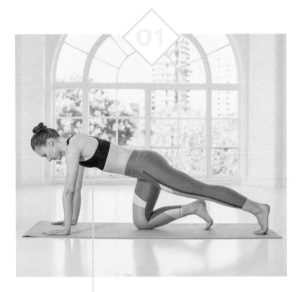

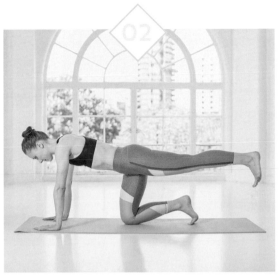

Set up your rib cage and hips as though you're trying to do a mini crunch, maintaining pressure in your stomach to keep you stable.

01. Start on all fours, making sure your back, neck and head make a straight line, and your chin is tucked in. Pull your shoulders back and down, so you've got tension under your armpits and ensure your elbow creases are pointing forward. Lengthen your left leg behind you, resting your toes on the back of the mat. Rock back slightly.

02. Raise your left leg off the floor so that it keeps that straight line with your head, neck and shoulders, and then drop it. Breathe out on the way up and in on the way down.

03. Repeat 20 times. Your right hand shouldn't be doing much, as the pressure will be on your right knee and left hand.

04. Reset to the start position then lengthen your right leg behind you and repeat the exercise.

CHILD'S POSE

01. Starting on all fours, rest your bottom on the heels of your feet, with your arms reaching forward and your toes pointed behind you.

02. Drop your head and breathe.

03. Hold for 30 seconds.

If your arms feel too tight, you can bend your elbows.

SQUATS 2.0

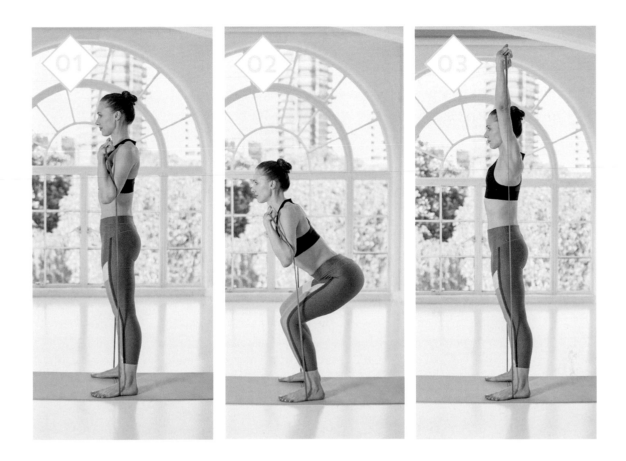

01. Step into a resistance loop band, keeping your feet hip-width apart and engaging your stomach by pulling the rib cage down. Make sure your chin is tucked in.

02. Squat as though you are sitting down. Be mindful as you go down that your chin and head don't go up or too low – don't round your body, keep your back straight.

03. Push up through the heels of your feet to standing, gripping the floor with your toes, and simultaneously raising your hands to the ceiling. Try to get your hands up so that your upper arm is in line with your ears.

04. Repeat 20 times.

THE 21-DAY FOOD PLAN

Diet is king when it comes to losing weight. My 21-day food programme is simple – there's no sugar, no alcohol and no fried food. But there is intermittent fasting, which gives your body time to reset. There's nothing new in the practice of fasting and, in fact, there have been studies investigating the potential positive effects as far back as the 1940s. Temporary abstinence is easier to stomach than total denial. I'm going to give you a simple and all-inclusive meal plan (see pages 100–101) which will show you what to eat over the next 3 weeks.

THERE ARE 3 TYPES OF DAY IN THIS PROGRAMME:

01/
FAST DAY
FOR 1 DAY A WEEK, YOU SHOULD EAT ONLY 500 CALORIES

Over the course of the 3 weeks, you will only have 3 days fasting. The 5:2 diet became a phenomenon in recent years but the problem for many people who have tried to restrict calories to this degree is how onerous the diet felt. It simply isn't feasible for a lot of people. One day a week is much easier to fit around an ordinary life. My 21-day programme incorporates the benefits of intermittent fasting with only half the hardship of the 5:2 diet.

During the fasting days, you will need to space out your food consumption to suit your body and needs. Some of us struggle to go without food in the morning, while others can cope with fasting until the evening, but cannot sleep on an empty stomach. In the recipe section (see pages 128–227), I have suggested meals that you can eat on a fast day. It's important to understand what 500 calories looks like. You don't want to waste calories eating something that is very calorific – you want to fill up on soups or vegetables, with some protein thrown in.

> **NB:** Intermittent fasting is not appropriate for everyone. Do not do this calorie-restricted day if you are pregnant, have a condition such as diabetes, or if you have suffered from an eating disorder. If you are on any kind of medication, please consult a doctor before undertaking the limited calorie day. Intermittent fasting is also not suitable for children, or those who are already very slim.

02/

16 HOURS OFF, 8 HOURS ON
FOR 5 DAYS YOU NEED TO EAT IN AN 8-HOUR WINDOW

What this means is you don't eat for the remaining 16 hours of the day. For example, from 8 o'clock in the evening until midday the next day you would go without food. This allows us to integrate intermittent fasting into your food plan. It's up to you how you decide to do it. You could eat breakfast at 8am and then stop eating at 4pm, or you eat a brunch at 10am and stop eating at 6pm, or you could simply eat a lunch and dinner. (There is no scientific evidence that suggests breakfast is a necessity. An exception to this are those people with impaired glucose regulation – if that's you, make sure you're starting the day with a good bowl of porridge.) It will be easiest if you stick to the same timings for the 5 days, otherwise you may find yourself with a long wait before you can eat again.

The 16 hour fast will give the digestive system a break. You do not need to calorie count on the non-fasting days. See page 98 for a suggested programme for the 21 days. You can move the days around – if you work weekends, you may prefer to change the day off, for example – or if you have a particularly tough Monday, you should move the 500-calorie day.

03/

DAY OFF
FOR 1 DAY A WEEK YOU CAN JUST EAT NORMALLY

There may be social reasons for needing a day off – it's not easy being the person at a birthday party or a dinner who feels they have to ask for a small portion – but it's also important to help you stick at the food plan over the 21 days. This isn't supposed to be an impossible struggle – you can do this programme and have a life, too. I'm a big believer in balance in life and diet, and it is important to have something to look forward to, and to be able to switch off a little from a strict regime.

You may be tempted to go crazy on this day at first and eat everything in sight. If you find yourself doing this, think about how this blowout makes you feel afterwards. Are you sluggish? Do you feel bloated? Does it actually make you feel good to be eating all this?

A FOOD DIARY FOR THE NEXT 21 DAYS

WEEK ONE						
MON	**TUES**	**WEDS**	**THURS**	**FRI**	**SAT**	**SUN**
Fast day – 500 calories	16 hours off, 8 hours on	16 hours off, 8 hours on	16 hours off, 8 hours on	16 hours off, 8 hours on	Day off	16 hours off, 8 hours on

WEEK TWO						
MON	**TUES**	**WEDS**	**THURS**	**FRI**	**SAT**	**SUN**
Fast day – 500 calories	16 hours off, 8 hours on	16 hours off, 8 hours on	16 hours off, 8 hours on	16 hours off, 8 hours on	Day off	16 hours off, 8 hours on

WEEK THREE						
MON	**TUES**	**WEDS**	**THURS**	**FRI**	**SAT**	**SUN**
Fast day – 500 calories	16 hours off, 8 hours on	16 hours off, 8 hours on	16 hours off, 8 hours on	16 hours off, 8 hours on	Day off	16 hours off, 8 hours on

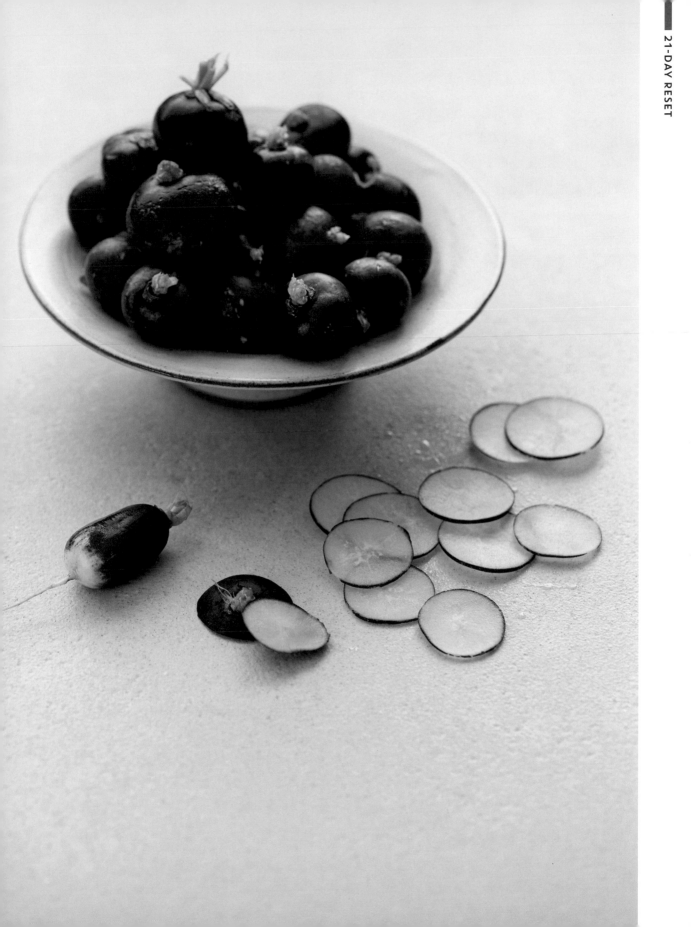

1 WEEK MEAL PLAN

This is a plan for your first week of meals. You can switch recipes around, but try to stay close to the total number of calories outlined here.

MONDAY

11am Breakfast		
Fast	Calories	0
	Fat (g)	0
	Carbs (g)	0
	Protein (g)	0

2pm Lunch		
Fast	Calories	0
	Fat (g)	0
	Carbs (g)	0
	Protein (g)	0

4pm Snack		
Fast	Calories	0
	Fat (g)	0
	Carbs (g)	0
	Protein (g)	0

7pm Dinner		
Italian Baked Sea Bass Page. 200	Calories	498
	Fat (g)	25
	Carbs (g)	16
	Protein (g)	47

Calories 498 / Fat (g) 25 / Carbs (g) 16 / Protein (g) 47

THURSDAY

11am Breakfast		
Date Porridge Page. 136	Calories	341
	Fat (g)	12
	Carbs (g)	54
	Protein (g)	10

2pm Lunch		
Chickpea Salad Page. 158	Calories	208
	Fat (g)	2
	Carbs (g)	39
	Protein (g)	9

4pm Snack		
Berry Protein Smoothie Page. 140	Calories	322
	Fat (g)	13
	Carbs (g)	45
	Protein (g)	7

7pm Dinner		
Baked Cod with Broccoli Page. 198	Calories	250
	Fat (g)	8
	Carbs (g)	18
	Protein (g)	26

Calories 1121 / Fat (g) 35 / Carbs (g) 156 / Protein (g) 52

FRIDAY

11am Breakfast		
Asparagus & Mushroom Omelette Page. 134	Calories	306
	Fat (g)	24
	Carbs (g)	7
	Protein (g)	17

2pm Lunch		
Gado Gado Page. 156	Calories	784
	Fat (g)	52
	Carbs (g)	60
	Protein (g)	35

4pm Snack		
3 Apricot & Coconut Balls Page. 222	Calories	207
	Fat (g)	12
	Carbs (g)	27
	Protein (g)	3

7pm Dinner		
Kung Pao Chicken with Courgette Pasta Page. 202	Calories	423
	Fat (g)	22
	Carbs (g)	17
	Protein (g)	28

Calories 1720 / Fat (g) 110 / Carbs (g) 111 / Protein (g) 83

TUESDAY

11am Breakfast Apple & Cinnamon Bircher Muesli Page. 138	Calories Fat (g) Carbs (g) Protein (g)	359 10 59 11
2pm Lunch Hoisin & Ginger Duck Salad Page. 172	Calories Fat (g) Carbs (g) Protein (g)	368 22 24 22
4pm Snack Skinny Chocolate Brownie Page. 212	Calories Fat (g) Carbs (g) Protein (g)	141 12 10 4
7pm Dinner Beef Tagliata Page. 171	Calories Fat (g) Carbs (g) Protein (g)	610 50 20 20

Calories 1478 / Fat (g) 94 / Carbs (g) 113 / Protein (g) 57

WEDNESDAY

11am Breakfast 2 x Egg Muffins Page. 147	Calories Fat (g) Carbs (g) Protein (g)	180 12 4 14
2pm Lunch Greek Couscous Salad Page. 164	Calories Fat (g) Carbs (g) Protein (g)	503 15 73 16
4pm Snack Salted Caramel Date Shake Page. 214	Calories Fat (g) Carbs (g) Protein (g)	189 2 64 2
7pm Dinner Asian Lettuce Burrito Page. 204	Calories Fat (g) Carbs (g) Protein (g)	348 22 21 21

Calories 1220 / Fat (g) 51 / Carbs (g) 162 / Protein (g) 53

SATURDAY

11am Breakfast Weetabix, Banana & Peanut Butter Shake Page. 141	Calories Fat (g) Carbs (g) Protein (g)	336 14 47 9
2pm Lunch Asian-style Tuna Tartare Page. 159	Calories Fat (g) Carbs (g) Protein (g)	263 13 6 30
4pm Snack Chia-Base Pizza Page. 152	Calories Fat (g) Carbs (g) Protein (g)	211 11 22 6
7pm Dinner Wrapped Salmon Page. 187	Calories Fat (g) Carbs (g) Protein (g)	378 23 12 31

Calories 1188 / Fat (g) 61 / Carbs (g) 87 / Protein (g) 76

SUNDAY

11am Breakfast Avocado on Toast Page. 146	Calories Fat (g) Carbs (g) Protein (g)	301 17 29 8
2pm Lunch Sea Bass Ceviche Page. 162	Calories Fat (g) Carbs (g) Protein (g)	361 17 17 35
4pm Snack Dairy-free White Chocolate Bark Page. 216	Calories Fat (g) Carbs (g) Protein (g)	300 27 17 3
7pm Dinner Garlic Chicken Page. 194	Calories Fat (g) Carbs (g) Protein (g)	732 24 57 77

Calories 1694 / Fat (g) 85 / Carbs (g) 120 / Protein (g) 123

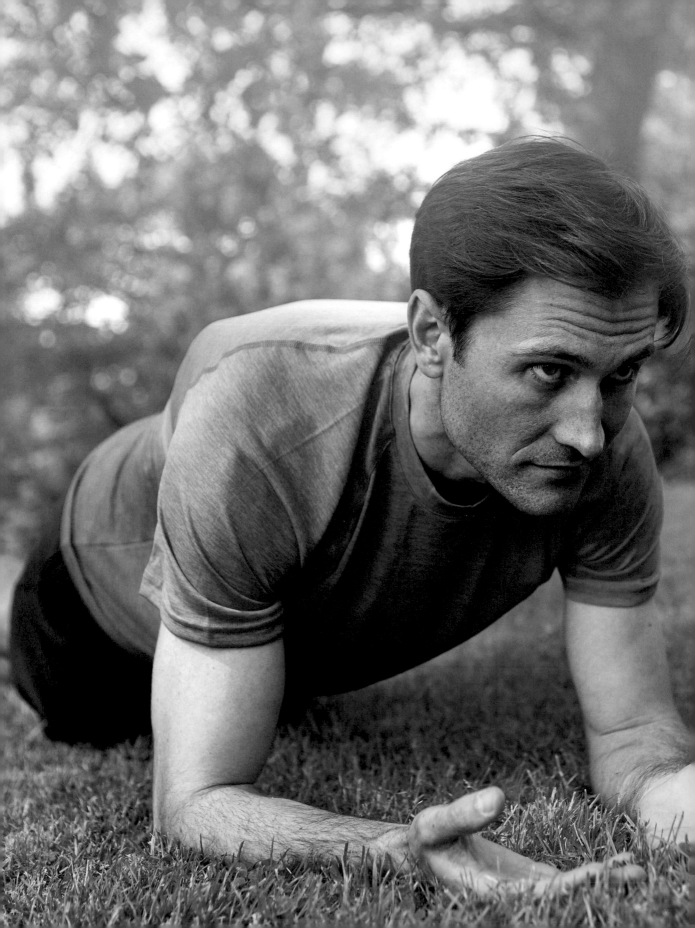

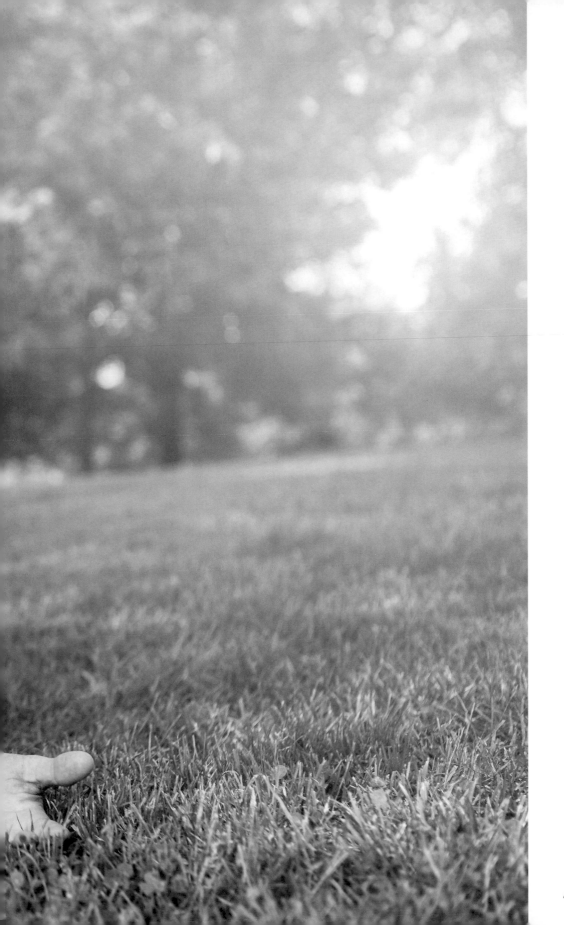

PART TWO

TRANSFORM

/12 WEEKS

Transformational Workout 1 – Weeks 4–16

- You will need a towel, an exercise mat, a foam roller, a mini loop band.
- Do the exercises barefoot.

Warm-up by doing the foam roller sequence set out on pages 234–241, followed by the Shoulder Warm-up on page 106.

EACH EXERCISE...

should be performed for 2 minutes. Follow the Golden Rules on page 60. The flow from one exercise into the other should be efficient but it does allow you to stop and reset your position when needed. As you get stronger, you will have to reset less and will therefore be able to perform a higher repetition count.

Once you've completed my 21-day Body Reset Programme, you'll be wondering what comes next. The answer is that you can now step up the exercise programme. You'll have changed the way your body moves and how you relate to it so now it's time to put those changes into action.

When you do these exercises, don't worry about the number of repetitions you do, but instead concentrate on doing them well. This is about the quality of the movement not the quantity. As you get stronger and fitter, you will be able to do more.

I have included 2 workouts to give you some variety. They are both all about 3 major moves of rotation, pushing and pulling. Do these exercises 5 times a week for 6 weeks once you have completed the 21-day Body Reset. In week 10, take a recovery week, and return to the exercises from week 3. Finally return to the Transformational Workout for the last 5 weeks.

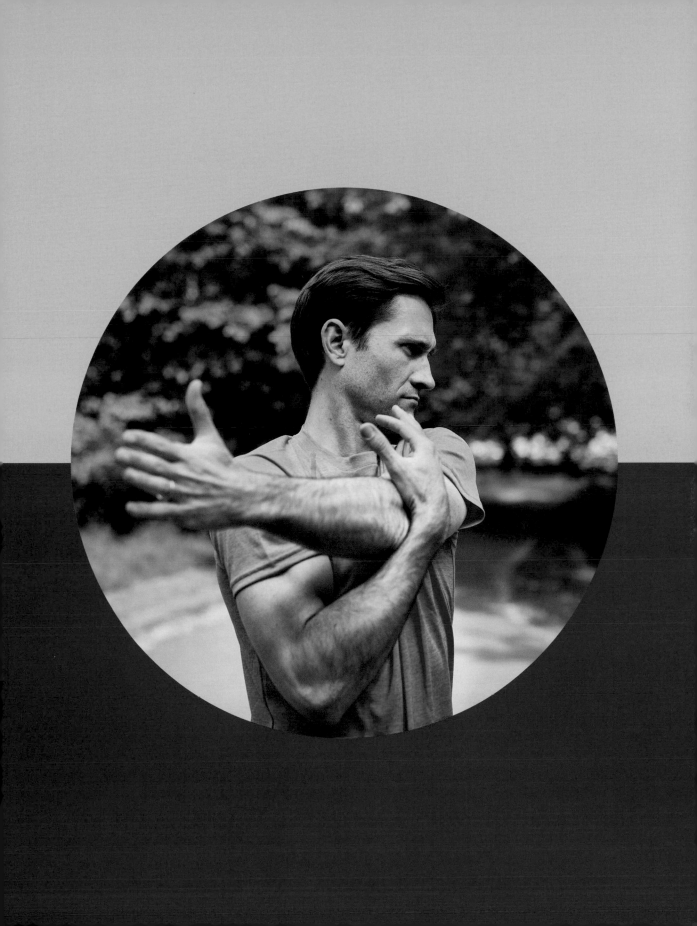

SHOULDER WARM-UP

01. Stand with your feet shoulder width apart. Wrap a resistance band around each hand. The movement tempo for each exercise is 1 – 0 – 1, which means 1 second open and 1 second close – with no pause in the middle.

Hold the band at chest height with your hands a little more than shoulder width apart.

Open your arms out to the side, squeezing your shoulder blades back and down. Maintain a brace in your core (stomach) and keep your rib cage down. You will naturally try to arch your back but fight against this by holding a tight core.

Return your hands to the starting position. Repeat 20 times.

02. Straighten your left arm down by your side. Focus on holding the left shoulder back and down. Imagine you are holding a rolled-up newspaper under that armpit, and don't let it go as you perform the next phase of the routine.

03. Raise your right hand up to the ceiling. As you do, try to pull your right shoulder blade back and down. Lower your arm down to your starting position. Repeat 20 times.

Repeat on the other side.

04. Hold your right arm up above your head (remembering to lock that shoulder blade back and down). Now raise your left arm up to chest height and return it to its original position beside you, with the new added move of opening the palm of your left hand. Find that rolled-up newspaper feeling again under your left armpit. Repeat 20 times.

Repeat on the other side.

05. Holding a good resistance on the band with your arms in front of you and keeping your shoulders back and down, raise your arms over your head.

06. Rotate your wrists, allow your shoulders to pull back and down, and keep those arms going around behind you until the band touches your butt. Maintain a constant resistance on the band throughout the movement.

As you improve you will be able to do this totally pain free. Once you can, increase the resistance of the band either by bringing your hand position closer together, or moving to the next strength of resistance band.

Return to your starting position and repeat.

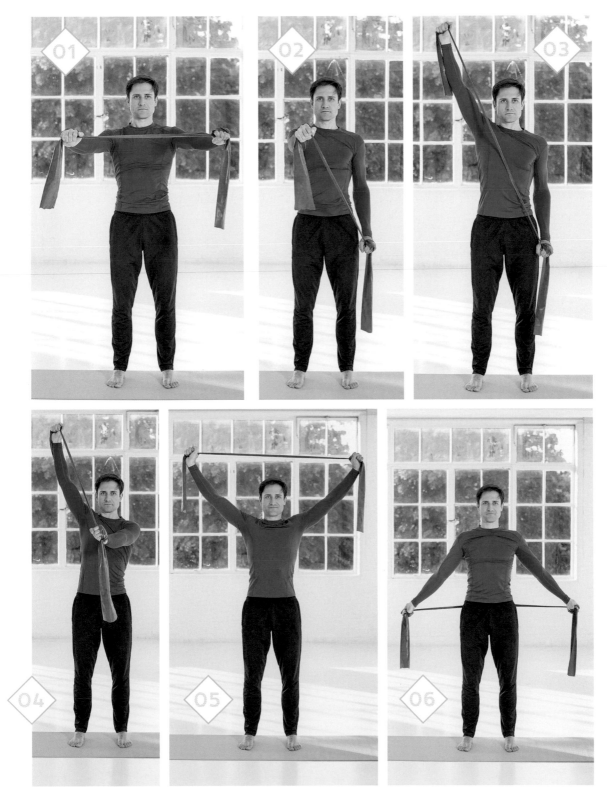

HIP BRIDGE

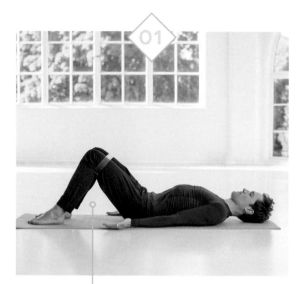

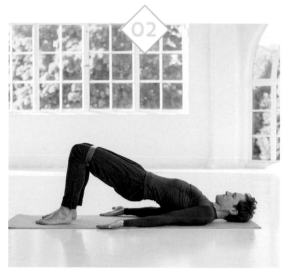

You can place a mini loop band around your knees, if you like. It will help you engage your glutes.

01. Lie on your back with your feet flat and your knees bent.

02. Lift your hips off the floor and hold them at the top for 3 seconds.

03. Lower your hips slowly.

04. Repeat for 2 minutes.

CLAMSHELL

01. Lie on your left side with your knees bent and your legs together. Place a mini loop band around your knees and rest your right hand on your right hip.

02. Keeping your feet together, lift your top knee, using your butt cheeks. Hold this position for 1 second then lower your knee.

03. Repeat for 2 minutes.

04. Repeat on the other side.

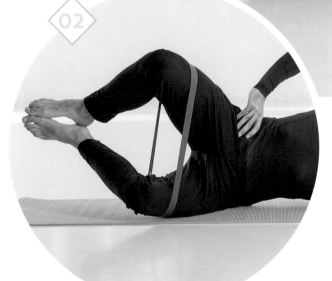

Rest your head on your left arm.

109

MINIBAND WALKS OF FAME

01. Stand with your feet apart and place a mini loop band around your knees.

02. Holding a squat position throughout the exercise, slowly 'crab' walk sideways from one end of the mat to the other. Maintaining a good tension on the mini loop band.

03. Continue for 2 minutes.

Hinge forward at the hips then bend your knees.

SIDE LUNGE

01. Stand with your feet hip width apart.

02. Take your right leg sideways. Lunge on to your repositioned leg until your knee is over your toe.

03. Push explosively back to the start position. Continue for 2 minutes.

04. Take your left leg sideways and repeat the exercise on this side. Continue for 2 minutes.

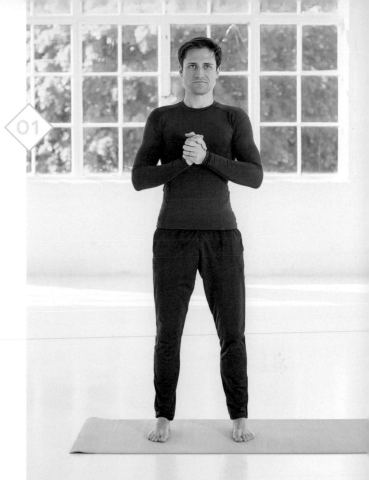

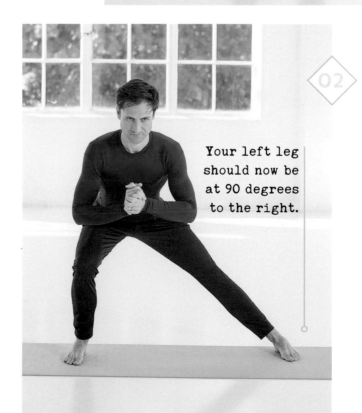

Your left leg should now be at 90 degrees to the right.

BOOTY LIFT

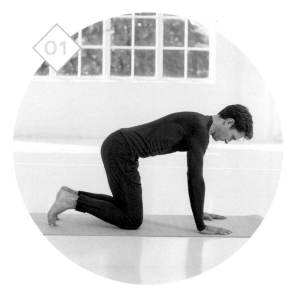

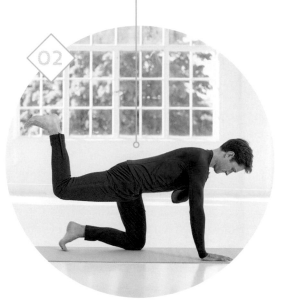

Keep your back straight.

01. Start on all fours, now lift off your left hand and place it on your chest.

02. Raise your right leg backwards, keeping your knee bent. Hold this for 1 second and then return to the start position. Continue this bent knee leg kick for 2 minutes.

03. Change sides and repeat.

FRONT PLANK

01. Resting on your elbows and toes, look down towards the mat.

02. Hold this position for 2 minutes.

Keep your body straight with your shoulder blades drawn back and down, abs braced and glutes tight.

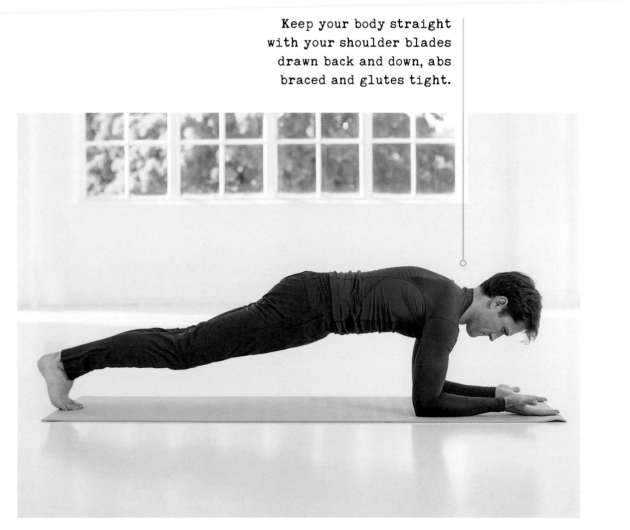

THE
CHEETAH

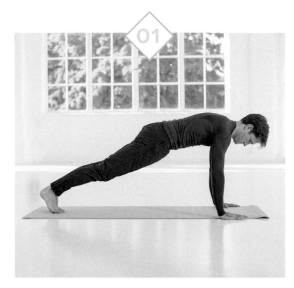

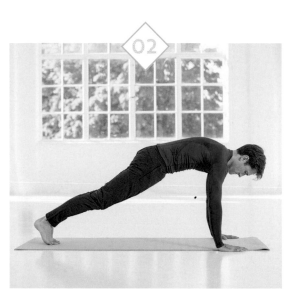

01. Start with both your hands and feet on the floor in a push-up position. Keeping your arms straight, allow your shoulder blades to come together slowly by allowing your chest to drop.

02. Hold this for 1 second then separate your shoulder blades as much as possible, keeping your spine straight.

03. Repeat for 2 minutes.

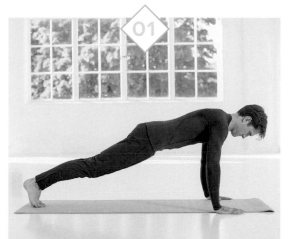

Push-up starting position.

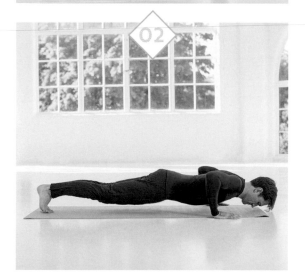

PUSH-UP & CHEAT PUSH-UP

The push-up and cheat push-up are the same exercise but the start position is different. With the cheat push-up you rest on your knees instead of your toes. Try to start with the push-up and as you get tired and begin to lose form, drop down into the cheat/kneeling position to complete the routine.

01. With your hands below your shoulders and your torso flat and straight, lower your hips/ chest until they are touching the floor.

02. Keep your body as straight as possible as you press up to the start position by extending your arms.

03. Repeat for 2 minutes.

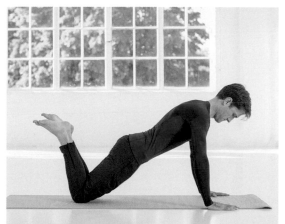

Cheat push-up starting position.

115

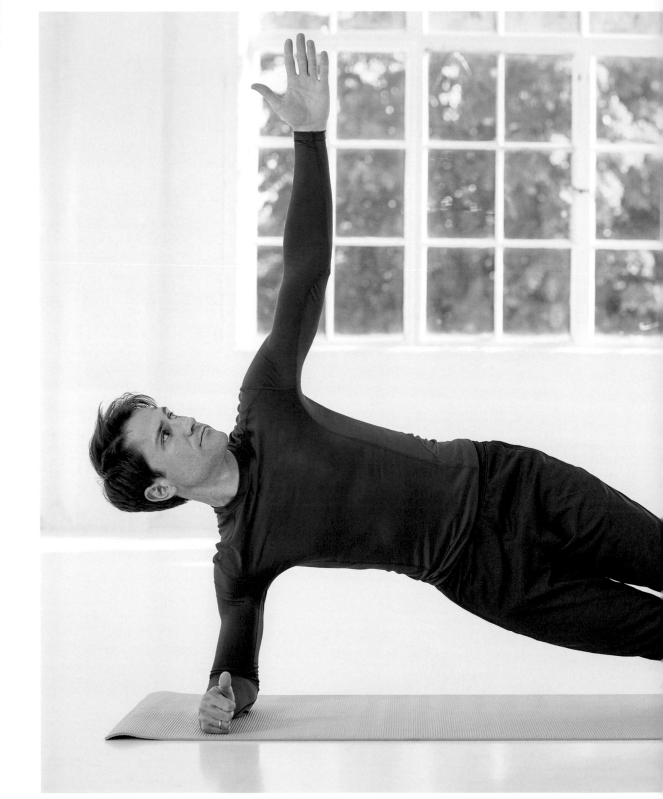

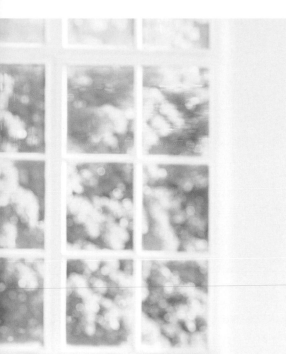

SIDE PLANK

01. Lie on your right side on the mat, resting on your right elbow and the sides of your feet.

02. Hold this position for 2 minutes.

03. Repeat on the other side.

Keep your body straight with your hips pushed forward, your abs braced and your glutes tight. Reach up with your left hand.

117

Transformational Workout 2

YOU WILL NEED

- A towel.
- An exercise mat.
- A foam roller.
- A medium tension resistance loop band.
- A step and a 2–3kg kettlebell (KB) or dumbbell. If you don't have one, use a 2kg bag of rice or a tin of paint instead.

Warm up by doing the foam roller sequence set out on pages 234–41, followed by the Shoulder Warm-up on page 106.

EACH EXERCISE...

should be performed for 2 minutes on each side. Follow the Golden Rules on page 60. The flow from one exercise into the other should be efficient but it does allow you to stop and reset your position. As you get stronger, you will have to reset less and will therefore be able to perform a higher repetition count.

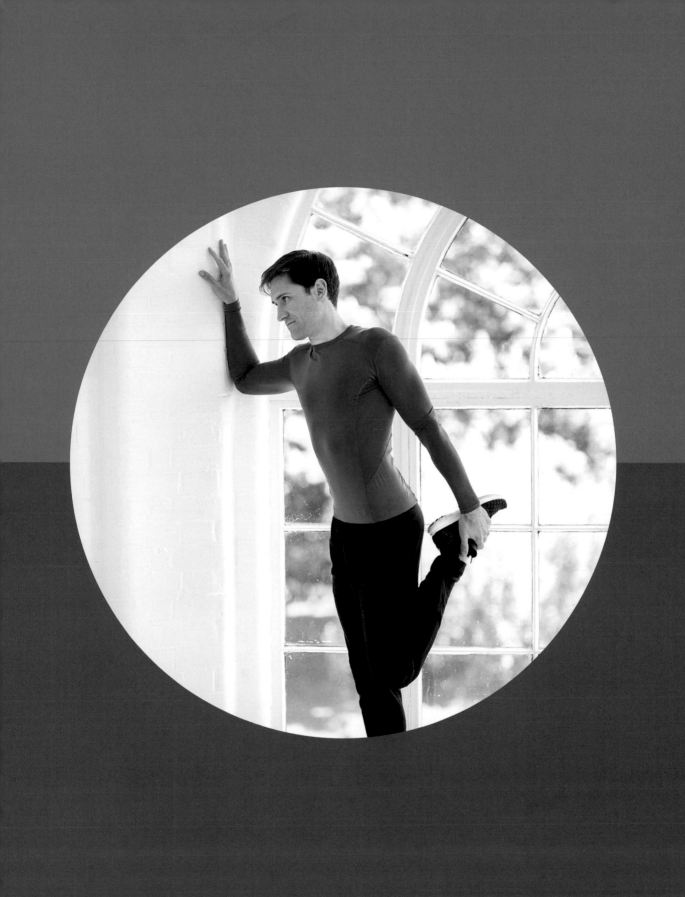

SUMO SQUAT

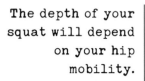

The depth of your squat will depend on your hip mobility.

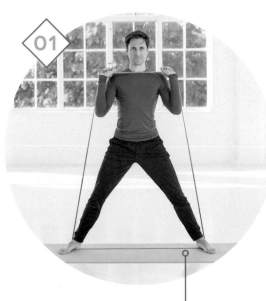

Grip the floor with your feet. Maintain a natural foot arch.

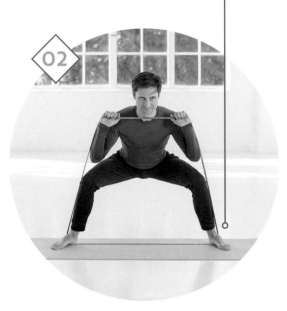

01. Step into a resistance loop band, standing with your feet wider apart than your shoulders, turning your feet so your toes are pointing out.

02. Squat down, making sure your knees stay over your toes.

03. Return to the starting position.

04. Repeat for 2 minutes.

RUSSIAN
STEP-UP

01. Hold the kettlebells or hand weights, pulling your shoulders back and down. Position the right foot on the step and step up.

02. Follow through with the left leg, raising your knee to hip height.

03. Not moving the stationary foot off the step, lower the left foot back down. Repeat for 1 minute, then continue on the other side.

Bring your knee to hip height.

TURKISH GETUPS

01. Lie on your back with your right knee bent and your right arm in the air holding the kettlebell.

02. Raise your upper body, bringing your weight to rest on your left hand and your right foot.

03. Shift your left knee to move under your hips and down until you are kneeling on this leg with your other foot flat on the floor. Your shoulder will need to rotate in the joint to keep the kettlebell above your head.

04. Laterally flex your spine so that your weight is no longer on your hand and your torso is erect. Rotate your shoulder.

05. Stand up, keeping the kettlebell above your head.

06. Reverse the steps until you are back lying flat on the floor.

07. Repeat for 2 minutes.

08. Swap the kettlebell into your other hand and repeat the process on the other side for 2 minutes.

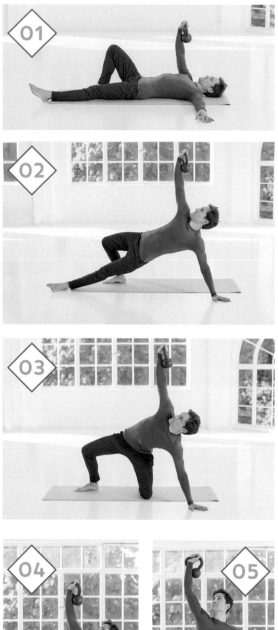

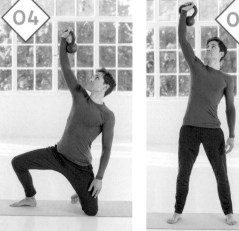

ALTERNATING SIDE PLANK

01. Start in the side plank position.

02. Place the top arm underneath your body and rotate so that the torso goes through 180 degrees.

03. Finish in the side plank position on the other side.

04. Repeat for 2 minutes.

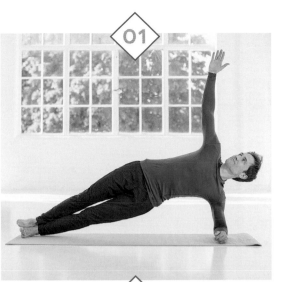

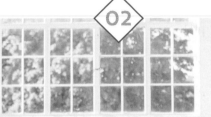

Keep your body straight, with hips pushed forward, abs braced and glutes tight throughout.

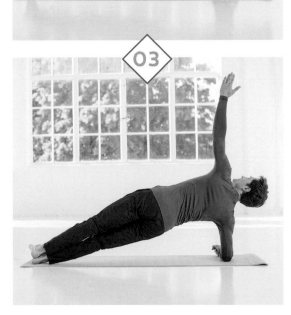

123

PRONE COBRA

01. Lie on your front with your arms outstretched in front of you.

02. Keeping your arms straight, take your hands out to the sides of your body, keeping them a couple of inches off the floor.

03. Repeat movement for 1 minute.

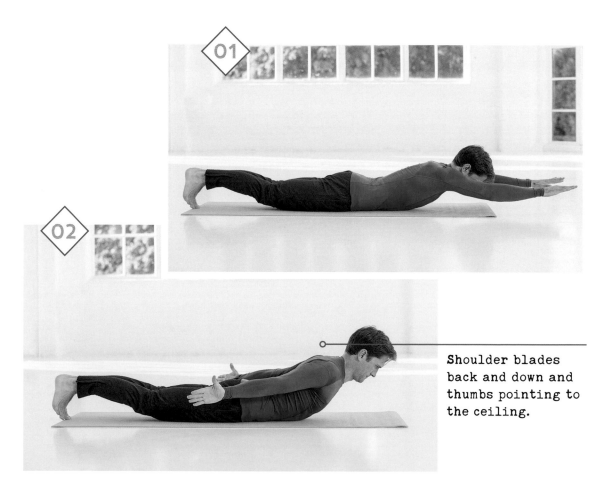

Shoulder blades back and down and thumbs pointing to the ceiling.

MAN OF STEEL

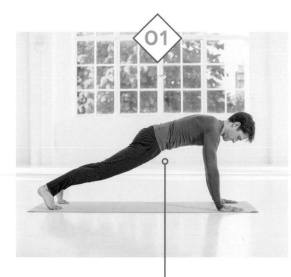

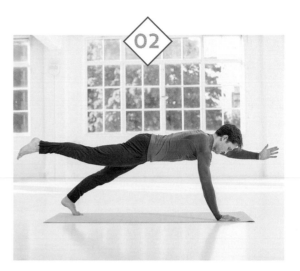

Keep your abs braced and your glutes tight.

01. Start in the push-up position. Keep your body straight with your shoulder blades drawn back and down,

02. Lift your right leg and left arm and keep them straight and level with your torso. Hold for 1 minute.

03. Reset to the start position and repeat the exercise with the opposite arm and leg. Hold for 1 minute.

KETTLEBELL PLANK ROW

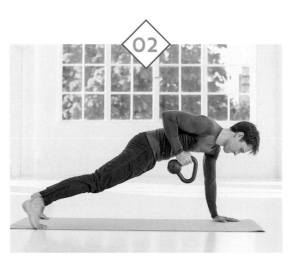

Keep your trunk stable and parallel with the floor.

01. Hold the kettlebell in one hand and assume the push-up position with your feet wide for balance.

02. Lift the kettlebell from the floor and row it back into the side of your body.

03. Lower the kettlebell slowly and repeat the lift.

04. Repeat for 2 minutes.

05. Reset to the start position then place the kettlebell in your other hand. Repeat the exercise for 2 minutes.

X MEN WALKS

01. Stand on the mat and place the resistance loop band under your feet. Lift the band up and cross it over to create an X.

02. Step one leg away, keeping your shoulders level, legs straight and trunk rigid, then bring the other leg to meet it. Walk sideways in this way to the edge of the mat. Step the other leg out to walk sideways to the opposite edge of the mat.

03. Continue for 2 minutes.

Hold the loop over your head with your hands shoulder width apart.

127

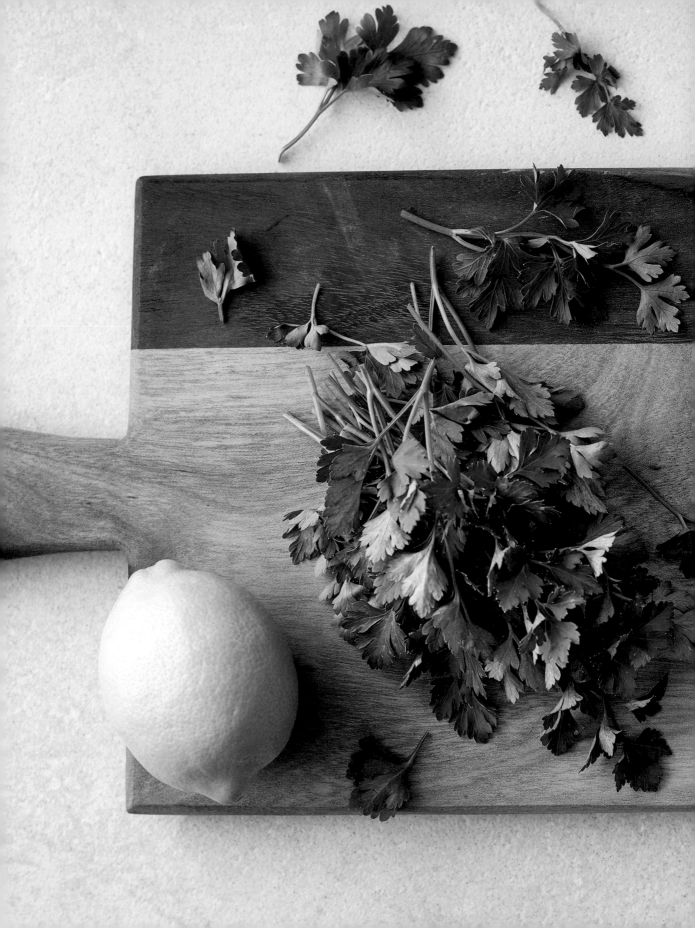

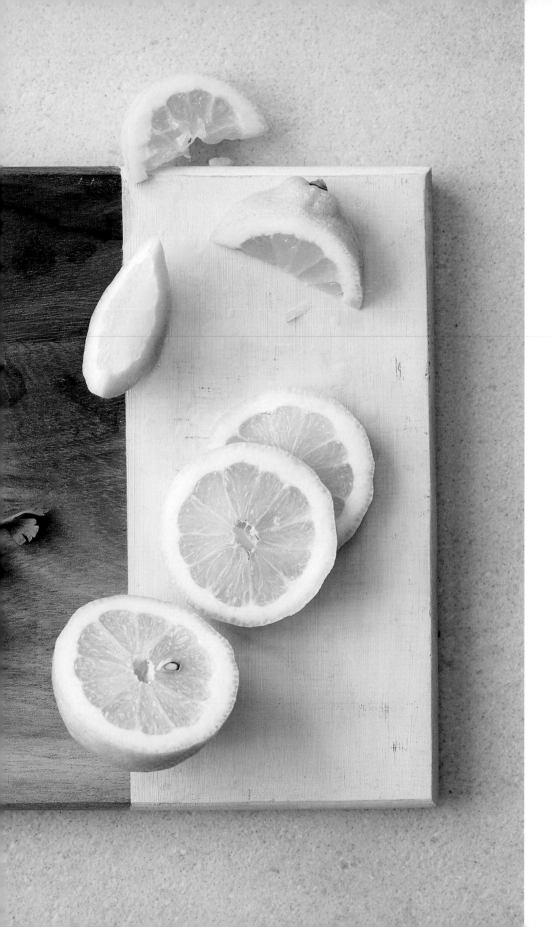

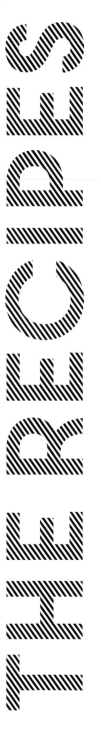

THE RECIPES

THE INSPIRATION BEHIND THE RECIPES

What does healthy eating look like? Lots of fresh vegetables, fish and organic food. And that's a thread running through my recipes.

It might help here to know what I eat on an average day. Breakfast might be a poached egg with avocado and cherry tomatoes, or smoked salmon for a treat if there's some in the fridge. I never eat cereal. I know it's easy but it is also frequently packed with sugar. For lunch, I might have a salad with either chicken and tuna. Dinner is usually meat or fish with vegetables (which might include potatoes). My diet is not difficult to replicate – and this is what I tell my clients to eat.

DIET BOGEYMEN?

I won't advocate anything faddy here – and this is certainly no exclusion diet where you cut out some food groups entirely. We have a habit of finding a dietary scapegoat to blame for the ills of the world (like obesity and heart disease). We fixate on 'good' and 'bad' foods. This isn't helpful.

An estimated 1 in 6 people in the UK have stopped eating bread and pasta regularly, in most cases because they've heard that gluten is bad for us. As a result, many people eat gluten-free versions, believing they are healthier. But gluten-free foods are sometimes highly processed and full of fat and sugar. And it's more like 1 in 100 people who really cannot tolerate gluten – they are coeliacs who suffer from a serious autoimmune disease. For everyone else, cutting out gluten may in fact be less healthy because you may not be consuming enough fibre, which is essential for good gut health.

Other people see the problem being dairy, or high-fat food, or sugar. The message is that if you avoid a particular 'poison' or if you 'eat clean', you will eliminate 'toxins' from your body. But there is no evidence to support this and our bodies are not actually overwhelmed by toxins. The current medical thinking focuses much more on gut health. It has been something of a neglected science in the past and now we're finally realising how much gut health affects the whole body.

Your intestines are home to most of the 100 trillion microbes that live in and on your body. It's like an ecosystem, consisting of organisms like fungi, bacteria, yeasts and protozoans. The bacteria in your gut break down your foods for you, produce vitamins and help train your immune system. My food plan is kind to your gut!

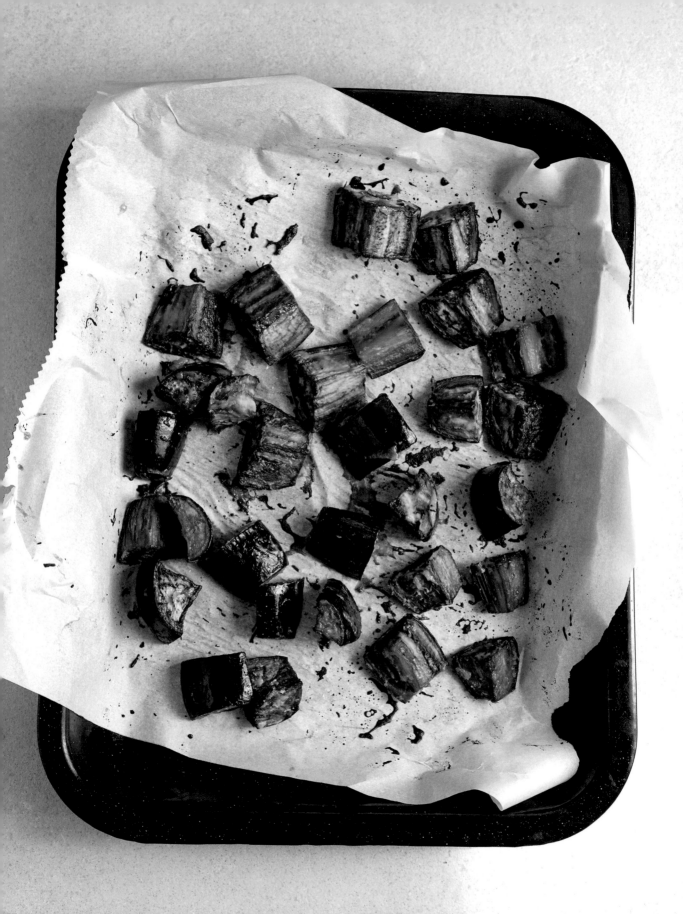

5 NUTRITION MYTHS AND THE REALITY

There's a lot of nonsense talked about nutrition. We all want miracle solutions that will make us slim and healthy – and that fact has created an appetite for the kind of information churned out on 'wellness' blogs, social media and even, occasionally, in newspapers. So, let's run through the food myths – and what the reality actually is.

MYTH 1

FAT MAKES YOU FAT

Low-fat diets have gone out of fashion in recent years but you still find some people peddling them as waistline shrinkers. Saturated fat has also been blamed for cardiovascular disease.

THE REALITY

Fat not only doesn't make you fat, but it is needed in your diet. I'm talking about the omega-3 and omega-6 fatty acids here that you can get from fish – not deep-fried crisps. It's good that fat's reputation has recovered from a dietary standpoint but make sure you're eating the right fats. As with most myths, there is a modicum of truth: do cut down or avoid trans fats, which have been shown to be bad for your health. You'll find trans fats in processed foods, including shop-bought sweets, cakes, biscuits and fried fast food.

MYTH 2

CARBS ARE THE ENEMY

Now that most people have stopped blaming fat for the ills of the world, they've found a new culprit – carbs. When it comes to the global obesity crisis, poor carbohydrates have now been identified as the sinner. You may have even tried a low-glycaemic diet yourself – swapping potatoes for lower GI sweet potatoes, for example. But the clinical evidence that these diets are healthier is inconclusive. They may make you grouchier, though – as anyone who's been in a relationship with someone carb-deprived can testify!

THE REALITY

Carbs usually aren't very filling and they're relatively high in calories, so it is easy to over-eat when you're chowing down on a bowl of pasta. So, the truth is that lowering your carb intake (especially the processed kinds) could help you lose weight – but this is only because it simply means you are eating less.

MYTH 3

YOU SHOULD EAT 'CLEAN'

Modern life has given us a new kind of guru: the clean eating queen (or king).

I don't want to sound too scathing here: wellness bloggers want us to be healthier, which is great. But 'clean eating' is actually a muddle of different ideas.

THE REALITY

What 'clean eating' diets do have in common is the fact that they're about avoiding certain food groups and this can create problems, leaving clean eaters deficient in certain nutrients. And there's the most extreme form of clean eating – a raw diet, which is touted as healthier because cooking 'denatures' nutrients. Just say no, kids. Cooking can actually help get nutrients out of veggies, because the heat breaks down the plant cell walls, releasing minerals for easier absorption.

The bigger problem here, as I see it, is that clean eating is an obsessive form of eating. I'm a big believer in enjoying your time on this earth – live a little! – and clean eating seems utterly joyless to me. Worse than that, it makes people divide foods up into 'good' and 'bad' and there aren't that many foods that fall into the 'good' camp – raw organic broccoli, perhaps?

Again, there's an element of clean eating that is correct: I also advise eating whole foods over processed foods but you don't need to start eyeballing raw kale smoothies.

MYTH 4

YOU NEED TO DETOX

The word detox is banned in this book. It is essentially clean eating squared. Companies promoting detoxes love to talk about 'toxins' and claim that detoxing clears poisons out of the body.

THE REALITY

If you were really ingesting poison, you would have a medical emergency on your hands. In which case, it would be even more important for you to be eating well, so you have the energy to recover! Your body already 'detoxes' itself – your organs, especially your liver and kidneys, filter out bad substances and excrete waste products. You can also make yourself sick through detox diets. There are much more successful ways to get healthy – starting with my programme!

MYTH 5

YOU NEED TO AVOID RED MEAT

The case against red meat is well known: it gives you cancer, goes the argument.

THE REALITY

The causes of cancer are complex. It is true that a study commissioned by the World Health Organisation in 2015 found that eating processed meat, such as bacon, corned beef or hot dogs, can raise the risk of suffering from bowel cancer, but experts think red meat, such as steak or lamb, is really a risk only for those who have an otherwise unhealthy lifestyle. It's far more important to quit smoking, get some exercise and eat your greens than to forgo a sizzling steak.

SERVES 1

This packs a protein punch and will keep you feeling full until your next meal. Eggs are one of the richest sources of protein and vitamins, including B12 (which helps keep your nervous system running well), vitamin D (which your body needs for absorbing calcium) and they also contain iodine (which the body needs to make thyroid hormones).

I know this is in the breakfast list, but it makes an easy lunch or dinner, too. Double the quantities if you're cooking for two.

ASPARAGUS & MUSHROOM OMELETTE

1 tbsp sunflower oil (or 4 sprays sunflower oil)

100g asparagus, trimmed

3 closed cup mushrooms, halved

2 medium free-range eggs

1 tbsp snipped fresh chives

sea salt and freshly ground black pepper

Place a griddle pan over a high heat and add half the sunflower oil.

Place the asparagus in the pan with the mushrooms and cook for 2–3 minutes on each side. Season with salt and pepper.

Meanwhile, whisk the eggs and place a frying pan over a medium heat.

Add the remaining oil to the frying pan and pour in the eggs. Stir until half cooked – the base should be firm but the top still runny.

Lower the temperature and add the cooked vegetables and the fresh chives.

Fold the omelette in half and cover the frying pan with a lid. Leave for 2 minutes, until cooked through.

TIP:
You can play around with the veggies you use – just make sure you adjust the cooking time appropriately.

// NUTRITION PER SERVING: CALORIES 306 / FAT 24G / CARBS 7G / PROTEIN 17G

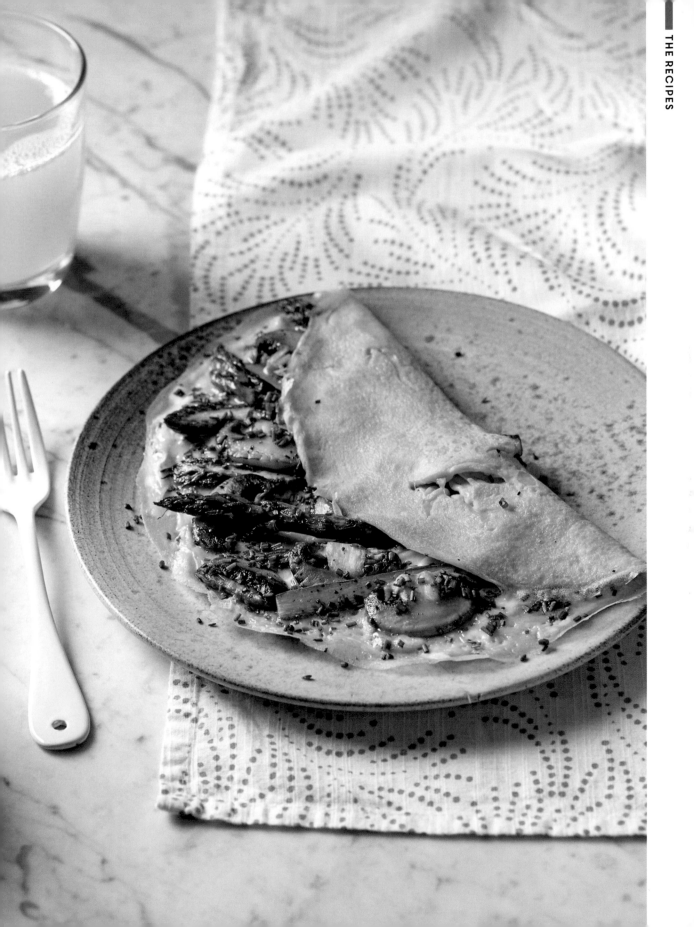

SERVES 1

Porridge is a hosanna to healthy living and it needn't take much time to make. Studies have shown that whole grains can lower blood pressure, promote healthy gut bacteria and even lower cholesterol. Add a sliced banana or ditch the toasted almonds and throw in some blueberries or blackberries - whatever floats your boat.

DATE PORRIDGE

500ml water
pinch of salt
2 Medjool dates, pitted
100g jumbo organic oats
a handful of flaked almonds,
    toasted (optional)

Measure the water, salt and dates into a blender and whizz until combined.

Place the oats in a bowl and pour the date mixture over the top.

Place in the microwave and cook for 2 minutes.

Stir the mixture, then return to the microwave for another 2 minutes.

Stir again, then set aside for 1 minute.

Sprinkle with the almonds and serve.

// NUTRITION PER SERVING: CALORIES 341 / FAT 12G / CARBS 54G / PROTEIN 10G

SERVES 6

According to food historians, shakshuka has Ottoman roots. It is certainly a dish that likes to travel - taking in North Africa, before spreading across the Middle East. It is particularly loved in Israel, where it has become a staple on breakfast menus. Perfect for a brunch when you're entertaining, it's warm, filling and kind to the waistline.

SHAKSHUKA

1 tbsp olive oil

1 medium onion, peeled and finely chopped

1 red pepper, deseeded and diced

2 garlic cloves, peeled and minced

1 tsp ground cumin

1 tsp paprika

1 tsp chilli flakes

2 tbsp red pepper purée

2 x 400g tins plum tomatoes

6 medium free-range eggs

a handful of fresh parsley leaves, roughly chopped

a handful of fresh coriander leaves, roughly chopped

sea salt and freshly ground black pepper

Place a cast-iron frying pan over a low to medium heat and add the oil.

Add the onion and a pinch of salt and cook for 15 minutes, until soft and lightly golden in colour. Add the red pepper and continue to cook for a further 5 minutes. Stir through the garlic and gently cook for another minute.

Mix the cumin, paprika and chilli flakes with a tablespoon of water and add to the pan. Cook for 1 minute to allow the oils to release. When the mixture is fragrant, stir in the red pepper purée and cook for another minute.

Add both tins of plum tomatoes and increase the heat, stirring every so often, until simmering. Check the seasoning and leave to simmer over a medium heat for 10–15 minutes. If the sauce starts to dry out, add a couple of tablespoons of water.

Finally, use the back of a spoon to create 6 'wells' in the sauce and crack an egg into each one.

Cover the pan with a lid and cook for a final 10 minutes, until the egg whites are cooked but the yolks are still runny.

Sprinkle the herbs over the dish before serving hot.

// NUTRITION PER SERVING: CALORIES 129 / FAT 7G / CARBS 10G / PROTEIN 7G

SERVES 1

This is the ultimate way to start the day on a healthy path and put some mojo into your morning. Muesli was invented in about 1900 by the Swiss physician Maximilian Bircher-Benner, who wanted to improve the health of his countrymen and women through their diet and was a big believer in the power of raw fruit and vegetables. Delicious and nutritious, this recipe is also dairy free.

APPLE & CINNAMON BIRCHER MUESLI

50g organic jumbo oats

1 tbsp mixed pumpkin and
   sunflower seeds

pinch of cinnamon

1 tbsp flaked almonds

½ apple, grated

125ml apple juice, plus a little
   water if needed

juice of ½ lemon

60ml nut or plant-based milk of
   your choice (or 2 tbsp
   coconut yoghurt)

1 tbsp fresh blueberries

Combine all the dry ingredients in a jar or bowl and cover with the grated apple, apple juice and lemon juice. If the mixture looks a little dry, stir through a dash of water. Cover and place in the fridge overnight.

In the morning, remove from the fridge and leave to stand for 10 minutes before adding the nut or plant-based milk or coconut yoghurt.

Top with the blueberries and tuck in.

// NUTRITION PER SERVING: CALORIES 359 / FAT 10G / CARBS 59G / PROTEIN 11G

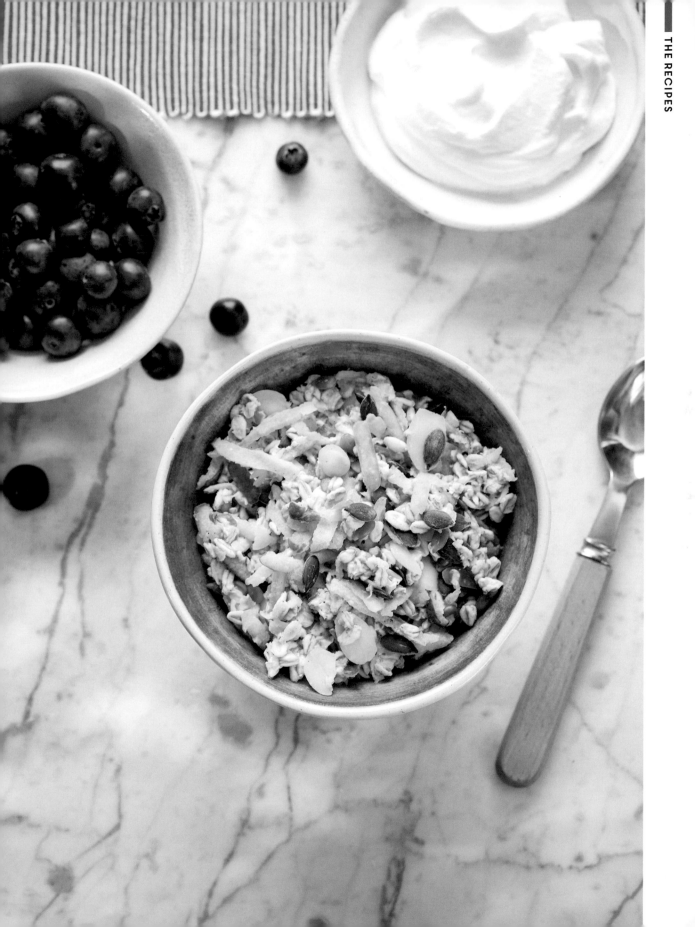

SERVES 1

Perfect as a post-workout pick-me-up as well as for breakfast. Prepare this the night before and then enjoy it as a small (healthy) reward. It is rich in antioxidants, which help protect the body from the harm caused by dangerous molecules called free radicals.

BERRY PROTEIN SMOOTHIE

50g oats

1 tbsp flaxseeds

6–8 unsalted almonds

50g mixed berries, blueberries, raspberries, strawberries or blackberries (frozen or fresh)

½ banana

240ml unsweetened almond milk or filtered water (or half and half)

Soak the oats, flaxseeds and almonds in water overnight.

Rinse and drain the oat mixture and place with all the other ingredients in a blender. Whizz for about 2 minutes until smooth. (You can add more nut milk if the smoothie is too thick.)

// NUTRITION PER SERVING: CALORIES 322 / FAT 12.6G / CARBS 45G / PROTEIN 7G

SERVES 1

When you want something fast and healthy as you run out the door in the morning, turn to this simple breakfast shake.

WEETABIX, BANANA & PEANUT BUTTER SHAKE

375ml almond milk

1 Weetabix

1 tsp vanilla extract

1 banana

1 heaped tbsp peanut butter

dash of sea salt

Measure all the ingredients into a blender and whizz until smooth and creamy.

Pour into a glass, or a flask if you're on the go, and enjoy.

From your chopping board to your table in 12 minutes
... These fritters will keep, so you can make them
early and reheat later. They're a good brunch dish
for a weekend when you're feeling lazy, too.

SPEEDY GREEN FRITTERS WITH AVOCADO & LIME 'BUTTER'

3 medium free-range eggs

4 tbsp buckwheat flour

100g courgettes, grated

100g broccoli, florets very finely chopped

30g fresh dill, finely chopped

50g feta, finely crumbled

splash of milk

1 tbsp rapeseed oil

1 avocado, peeled, destoned and chopped

juice of 2 limes

2 green chillies, deseeded and finely sliced (optional)

Combine the eggs and buckwheat flour in a large bowl. Whisk until combined.

Squeeze the moisture out of the courgettes.

Add the courgettes, broccoli, dill and feta to the bowl and mix well. Loosen the mixture with a splash of milk.

Place a large non-stick frying pan over a high heat and add the oil.

Put 3 large serving spoons of the vegetable mixture into the pan to make 3 fritters. Turn the heat down to medium and cook for 3–4 minutes, until the fritters are solid enough for you to flip them over. They should be golden brown on the underside. Leave to cook and become golden on the other side, then remove from the pan and keep warm. Repeat to make 3 more fritters (there is no need to add any more oil to the pan after the first batch).

Meanwhile, using a hand blender, blend the avocado with the lime, then add the chilli, if using.

Serve the fritters with the avocado and lime 'butter' on top.

// NUTRITION PER SERVING: CALORIES 162 / FAT 12G / CARBS 9G / PROTEIN 7G

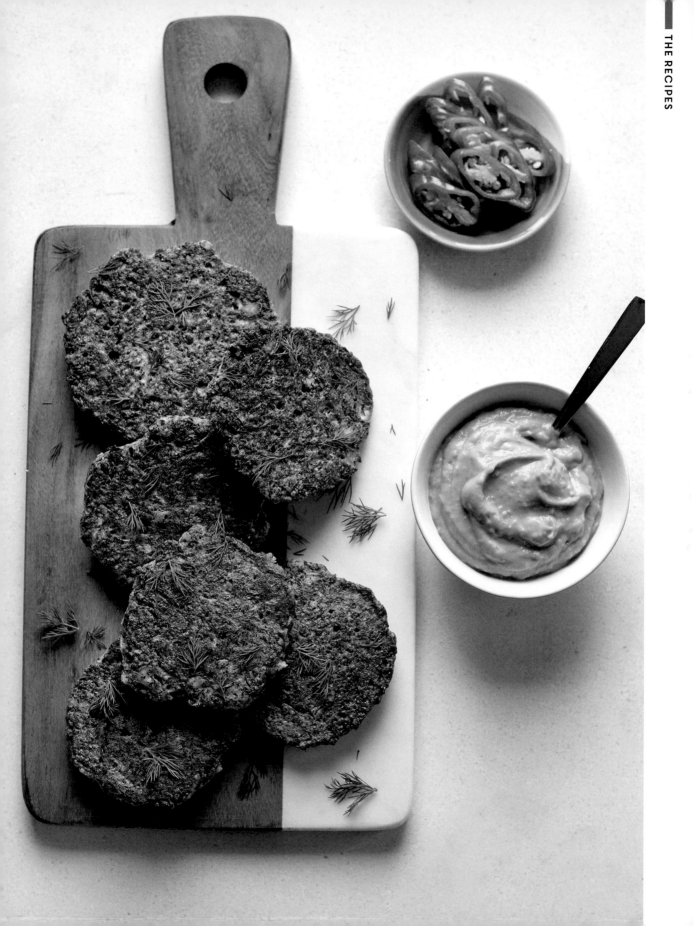

SERVES 1

A triple breakfast treat that's a great alternative to a fry-up. The egg will give you a protein boost, the avocado is rich with vitamin E and healthy fats, while the mushroom is a good source of selenium, which helps thyroid function. You can boil the eggs if you prefer.

POACHED EGG, AVOCADO & PORTOBELLO STACK

1 large Portobello mushroom, cleaned thoroughly
1 tsp coconut oil
1 egg
½ avocado, peeled, destoned and sliced
1 lemon wedge
sea salt and freshly ground black pepper
a few basil leaves, to garnish

Preheat the grill to medium-high.

Remove the stem of the mushroom and brush the coconut oil over the cap of the mushroom. Season it with salt and pepper. Place the mushroom under the grill and cook for 6 minutes (check if it is done after 4 minutes).

Meanwhile, poach or boil the egg.

Remove the mushroom from the grill and place on a plate.

Layer the avocado on top and squeeze over some lemon juice.

Top with the egg and season with pepper and basil before serving.

// NUTRITION PER SERVING: CALORIES 266 / FAT 20G / CARBS 15G / PROTEIN 11G

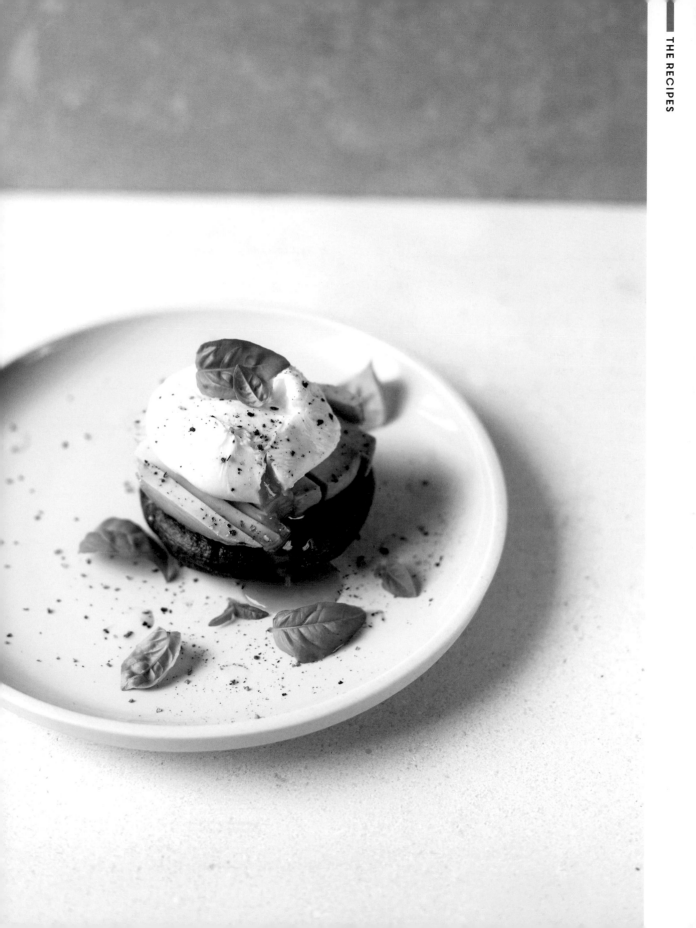

No recipe book (or British brunch menu) would be complete without avocado on toast these days, would it? Super quick, ultra easy and as tasty a breakfast as can be, this is my simple take on a modern classic.

AVOCADO ON TOAST

½ avocado, peeled and destoned
1 slice of your favourite
  wholegrain bread
juice of ¼ lemon
pinch of chilli flakes (optional)
feta (optional)
sea salt and freshly ground black
  pepper

Mash the avocado. Toast the bread then spread with avocado.

Season with a pinch of salt and pepper and a squeeze of lemon.

Sprinkle with chilli flakes and feta, if using, and serve.

// NUTRITION PER SERVING (WITHOUT FETA): CALORIES 301 / FAT 17G / CARBS 29G / PROTEIN 8G

MAKES 12

How do you like your eggs in the morning? How about as a muffin? Forget the egg muffins from a famous food chain, these are far healthier and tastier, too. You can make them in advance and keep them in the fridge. Halve the ingredients to make 6.

EGG MUFFINS

40g asparagus, trimmed and finely chopped

40g chestnut mushrooms, finely chopped

40g red peppers, deseeded and finely chopped

1 red onion, peeled and finely chopped

1 tbsp olive oil, plus extra to grease

12 medium free-range eggs

60g ricotta

6 small vine tomatoes, quartered or halved

40g fresh spinach, washed and roughly chopped

a handful of fresh parsley leaves, roughly chopped

sea salt and freshly ground black pepper

Preheat the oven to 200°C/Fan 180°C and lightly grease a 12-hole muffin tin with olive oil.

Place the asparagus, mushrooms, peppers and onions in a bowl with the oil and season with a generous pinch of salt and pepper. Mix well with your hands, making sure that all the vegetables are well coated. Tip into a roasting tin and place in the oven for 5 minutes.

Remove and leave to cool slightly.

Meanwhile, beat the eggs together in a large bowl.

Place a teaspoon of ricotta and half a tomato in each of the muffin cups, then pour over some of the beaten eggs, half filling each of the cups.

Divide the roasted vegetables, spinach and parsley between the cups, then pour over the remaining eggs.

Bake in the oven for 15–20 minutes, until the muffins are just set and golden brown.

Remove from the oven and leave to cool for a few minutes in the tin before turning out on to a cooling rack.

// NUTRITION PER SERVING: CALORIES 90 / FAT 6G / CARBS 2G / PROTEIN 7G

SERVES 2

A mid-week treat that not only uses up the weekend leftovers in the fridge but is also a delicious way to get the kids to eat their veggies.

VEGETABLE ROSTI WITH SMOKED SALMON

1 large baking potato

1 carrot

1 medium free-range egg, beaten

pinch of sea salt and freshly ground black pepper

1 tbsp olive oil

100g smoked salmon, sliced

FOR THE TOPPING

60g cream cheese

a small handful of fresh flat-leaf parsley

½ tbsp fresh lemon juice

Scrub the potato and carrot, then place them in a saucepan of boiling water over a medium heat. Parboil the carrot for 5 minutes, then remove it from the pan. Continue to cook the potato for a further 5 minutes, then remove it from the pan.

Set them both aside to cool and dry out, preferably overnight. In the morning, grate the potato and carrot on a coarse setting into a large bowl.

Mix in the egg and seasoning.

Place the oil in a large frying pan over a medium heat, then put 1 tablespoon of the vegetable mixture into the pan and flatten with a spoon. Place another 3 small rounds in the pan, making sure they are well spaced. Cook for 4–5 minutes on each side, until golden brown.

Meanwhile, to make the topping, put the cream cheese, parsley and lemon juice into a blender and pulse several times, until well mixed together.

To serve, divide the rosti and smoked salmon between 2 plates and top with a dollop of the cream cheese sauce.

// NUTRITION PER SERVING: CALORIES 191 / FAT 13G / CARBS 10G / PROTEIN 10G

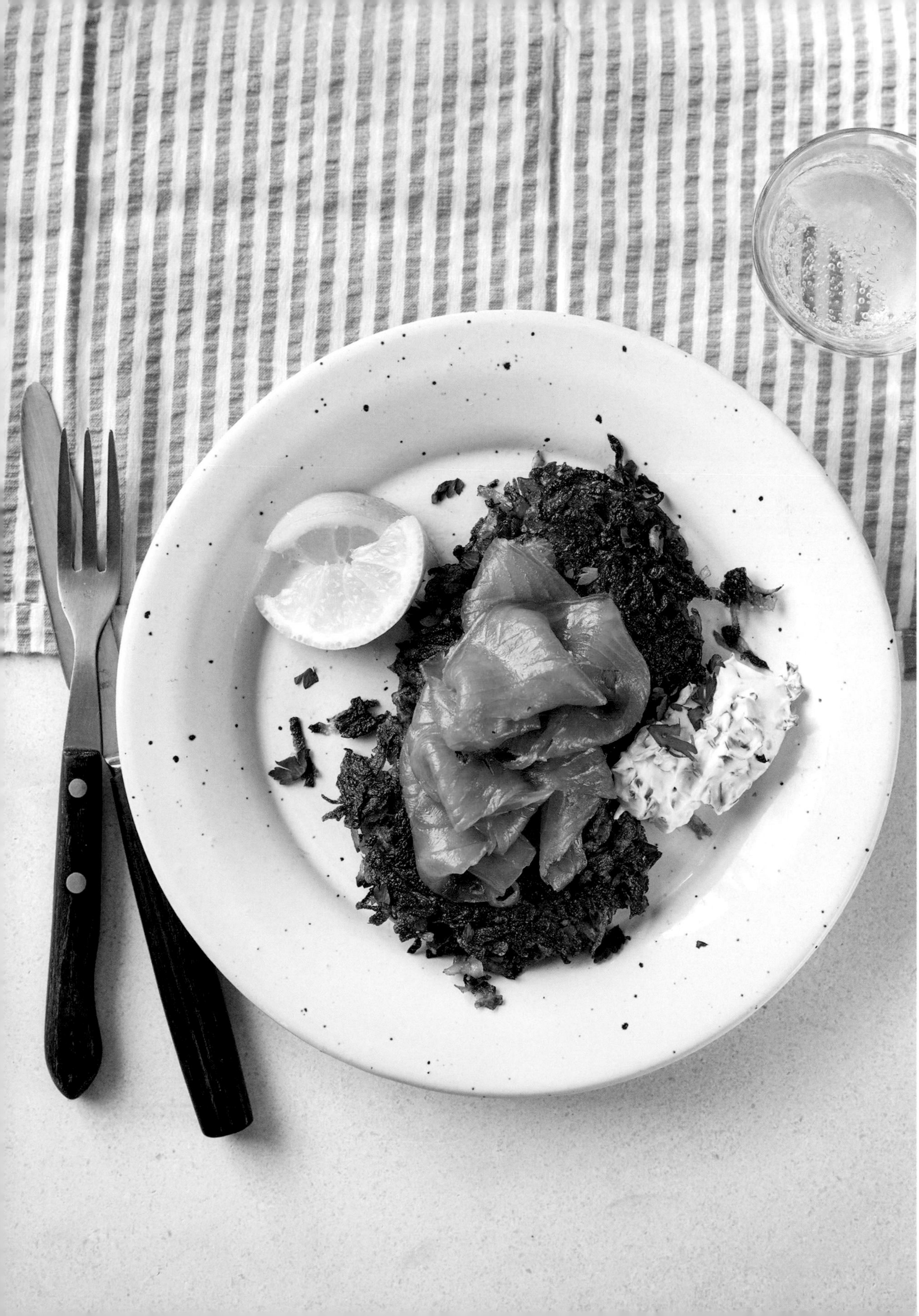

The breakfast equivalent of a cold shower, this will wake you up with a ginger tingle.

WAKE-UP-WORLD CARROT, APPLE & GINGER JUICE

6 carrots, peeled

4 apples, peeled and cored

5cm piece fresh root ginger,
   peeled and diced

juice of ½ lemon

Whizz all the ingredients in a blender or juicer, until smooth.

Pour into a glass and serve.

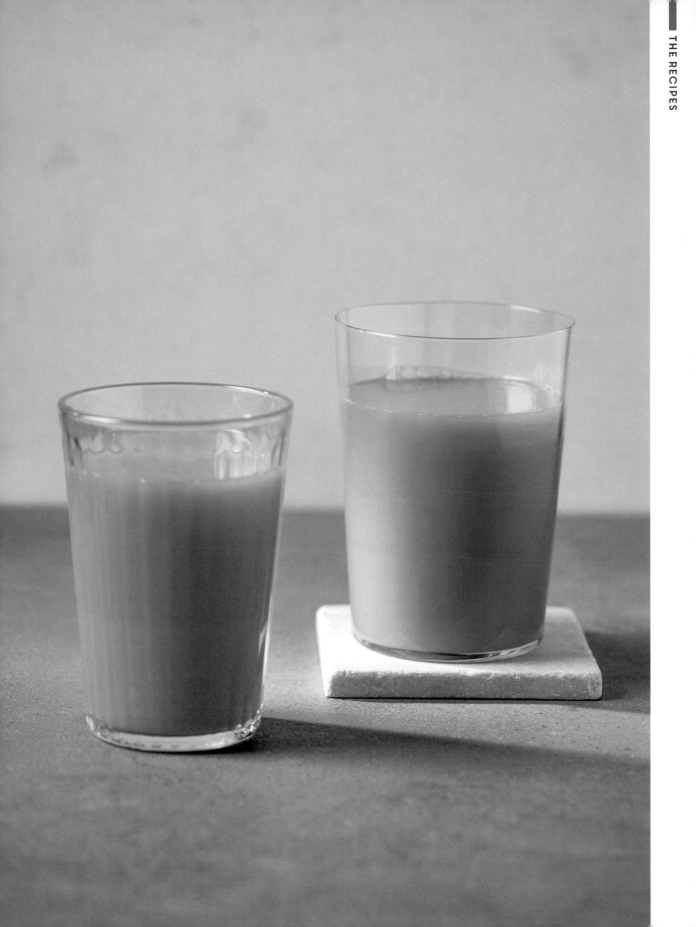

Think there's no way you can enjoy pizza when you're on a health kick? Think again. It's a long way from your favourite take-away pizza, but I promise you'll love it - and it's a fun recipe to make with the kids, too. It's also cheese-free, so it's a pizza that vegans can tuck into . . .

CHIA-BASE PIZZA

1½ tbsp olive oil, plus extra for greasing

1 onion, peeled and finely chopped

1 garlic clove, peeled and finely chopped

pinch of chilli flakes

1 tsp tomato purée

1 x 400g tin plum tomatoes

3 tbsp chia seed powder

80ml water

200g ground almonds

a handful of fresh porcini mushrooms, roughly chopped

12 black olives, sliced

a handful of rocket

a small bunch of fresh oregano

sea salt and freshly ground black pepper

Start by making a quick tomato sauce. Place a saucepan over a medium heat and add 1 tablespoon of the oil. Once hot, add the onions and a pinch of salt and cover the pan with a lid. Cook for 10–15 minutes, until the onions are soft and have a little colour. Add the garlic and chilli flakes and cook for 1 minute.

Stir through the tomato purée and cook for a further minute before adding the plum tomatoes. Turn down the heat and leave to simmer and reduce while making the rest of the pizza.

Preheat the oven to 220°C/Fan 200°C and line a baking tray with baking paper.

Measure the chia seeds into a small bowl, add the water and leave to soak for 10 minutes.

Mix the ground almonds and a pinch of salt in a separate bowl and season with pepper. Add the soaked chia and mix together with your hands until a dough forms.

Brush the baking paper on the tray lightly with oil and place the ball of dough in the middle. Cover it with another piece of baking paper and press down to make a flat pizza base, about 5mm thick all the way around. Discard the top piece of baking paper.

Bake in the oven for 12–15 minutes, until the surface starts to colour.

// NUTRITION PER SERVING: CALORIES 211 / FAT 11G / CARBS 22G / PROTEIN 6G

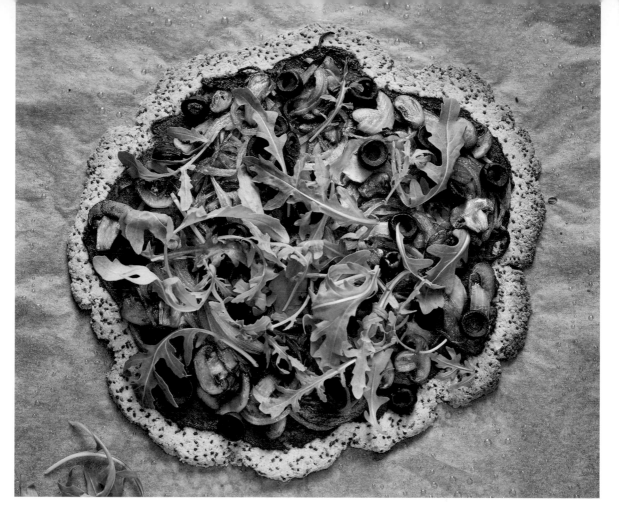

While the base is cooking, put the remaining oil in a frying pan over a medium heat and add the mushrooms and a generous pinch of salt and pepper.

Remove the base from the oven but keep it on its tray. Spoon tomato sauce over the base, leaving 1cm uncovered all the way around for the crust.

Top the sauce with the mushrooms and olives.

Return the pizza to the oven to bake for another 7–10 minutes.

Remove from the oven and finish with the rocket and a few oregano leaves.

SERVES 2

Did you know that 75 per cent of Japanese people consume miso soup at least once a day (it gets served for breakfast, lunch and dinner . . .)? It's the ultimate comfort food – and fermented foods can be packed with beneficial bacteria, too.

MISO FISH SOUP

30g instant miso soup powder

400ml water

50g shiitake mushrooms, stalks removed

1cm piece fresh root ginger, peeled and crushed

60g rice noodles

½ tbsp tamari (Japanese gluten-free soy sauce)

100g skinless white fish of your choice, cut into cubes

100g pak choi, shredded

a small handful of fresh coriander leaves

2 spring onions, trimmed and sliced

Put the miso powder into a blender with the water and run on high for 10 seconds.

Add the mushrooms and blend on and off 2–3 times, until they are roughly chopped.

Transfer into a saucepan and add the ginger, noodles, tamari and fish. Place over a medium heat and simmer for 3 minutes, then add the pak choi and simmer for another minute.

Remove from the heat and sprinkle with the coriander leaves and spring onions to serve.

// NUTRITION PER SERVING: CALORIES 321 / FAT 7G / CARBS 34G / PROTEIN 30G

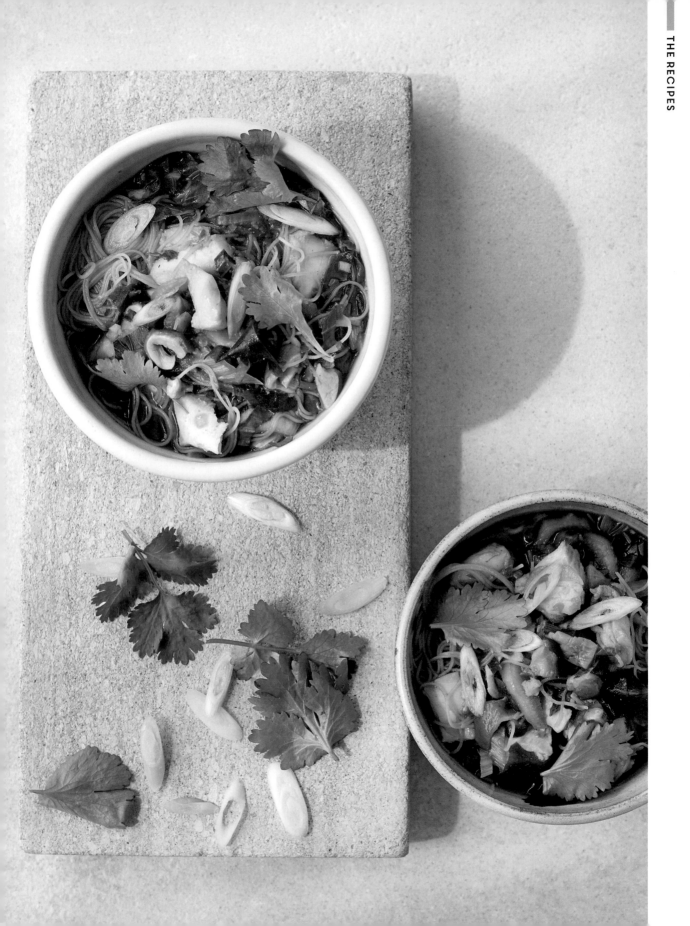

This is my take on an Indonesian salad - crunchy, zingy and delicious. 'Gado Gado' means 'mix mix' because people chuck in whatever veggies are in season. Feel free to play around with the ingredients and find out what you most enjoy. If you pack the peanut sauce in a little container on the side, you can take this dish into work for lunch.

GADO GADO

1 tbsp sesame oil

200g carrots, peeled and cut into matchsticks

8 baby corn, chopped

2 pak choi, chopped

300g beansprouts

PEANUT SAUCE

125g roasted unsalted peanuts

1 tbsp fish sauce

juice of ½ lime

2 tbsp sunflower oil

1 garlic clove, peeled

½ tsp chilli powder

1 tsp honey

pinch of salt

Put all the sauce ingredients into a blender with 150ml water and whizz on high speed for 1 minute. Set aside.

Place the sesame oil in a large wok over a high heat. Add the carrots, baby corn and pak choi and stir-fry for 3 minutes.

Once the vegetables begin to soften, add the beansprouts and continue to stir-fry for a further 2 minutes.

Drizzle the peanut sauce over the top and serve immediately.

// NUTRITION PER SERVING: CALORIES 784 / FAT 52G / CARBS 60G / PROTEIN 35G

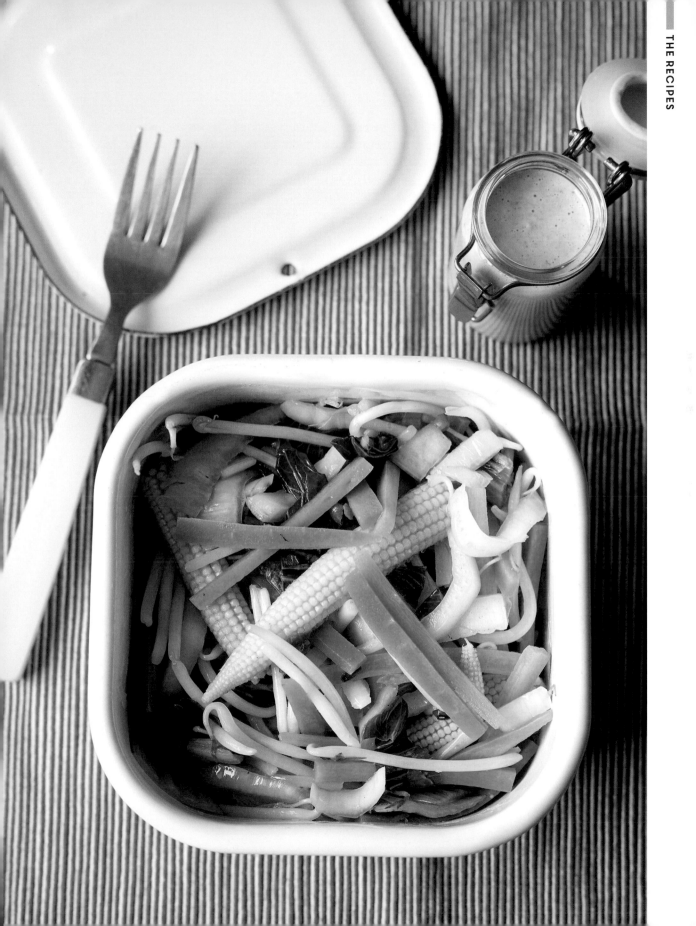

SERVES 1

A light vegan salad that you can make in 5 minutes in the evening, box up and take to work the next day. It makes a good addition to a summer buffet, picnic or barbecue, too.

CHICKPEA SALAD

1 red pepper, deseeded and
  chopped
2 celery sticks, chopped
2 carrots, peeled and grated
100g chickpeas (from a jar, ideally)
small bunch watercress, chopped
small bunch fresh mint, chopped
juice of ½ lemon
sea salt and freshly ground black
  pepper

Combine the pepper, celery, carrots, chickpeas, watercress and mint in a large bowl.

Dress with lemon juice and season with salt and pepper.

// NUTRITION PER SERVING: CALORIES 208 / FAT 2G / CARBS 39G / PROTEIN 9G

SERVES 4

If you can afford it, try to get your hands on some fresh, sustainable tuna that looks purply pink and glossy. It should have that familiar, fresh smell of the sea. It will be heaven, I can promise you. This dish is also nature's internal moisturiser - the tuna is packed with omega-3 fatty acids that give you great skin, while avocado is also full of healthy oils.

ASIAN-STYLE TUNA TARTARE

2 x 250g sushi-grade tuna steaks

1 tbsp sesame seeds

2 tbsp sesame oil

2 tbsp fresh lemon juice

½ red onion, peeled and finely chopped

1 avocado, peeled, destoned and cubed

1 tbsp soy sauce

a handful of fresh coriander leaves, finely chopped

pinch dried chilli flakes

Finely chop the tuna and place in a bowl.

Add the remaining ingredients and mix well.

Divide between 4 plates and serve.

SERVES 2

I think watercress is massively underrated. It's great in salads and sauces - but best of all in soup. This is a real warmer on a winter's day.

WATERCRESS SOUP

2 tbsp olive oil

2 banana shallots, peeled and roughly chopped

1 leek (the white part only), washed and roughly chopped

1 celery stick, roughly chopped

500ml chicken stock (I recommend Truefoods or use homemade stock or stock cubes)

100g watercress, washed and roughly chopped

80g baby leaf spinach, washed

sea salt and freshly ground black pepper

Place a saucepan over a medium heat and add the oil, shallots, leek and celery. Sweat, without colouring, for 4 minutes, stirring occasionally to stop the vegetables sticking.

Pour in the stock and bring up to the boil. Turn down the heat and leave to simmer for 3 minutes.

Add the watercress and spinach and simmer for another minute.

Remove from the heat, transfer the entire contents of the pan into a blender and whizz until smooth.

Season with salt and pepper to serve.

// NUTRITION PER SERVING: CALORIES 144 / FAT 14G / CARBS 6G / PROTEIN 3G

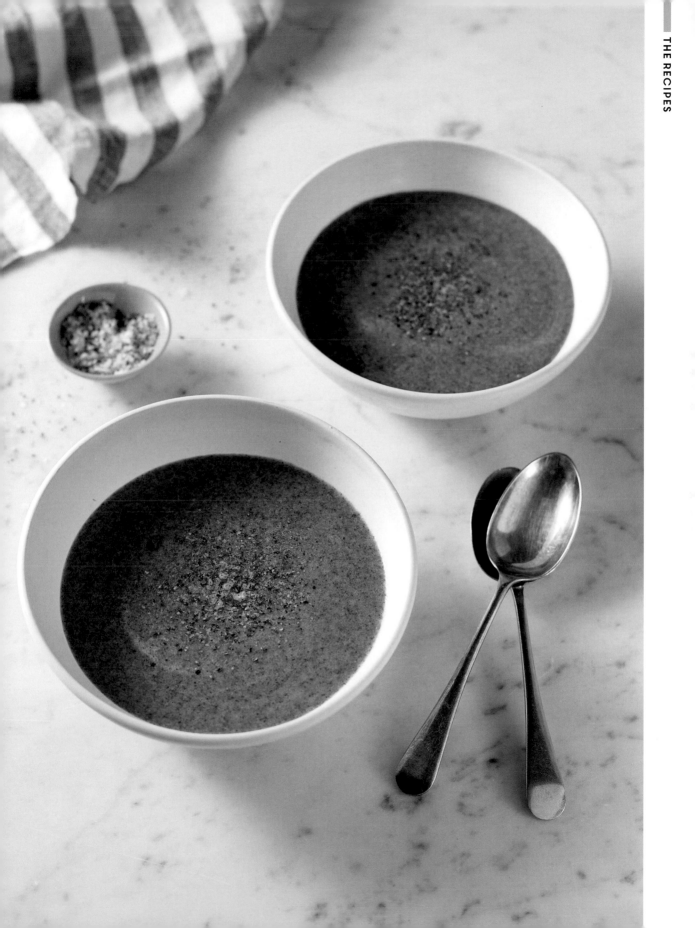

Ceviche is considered a national dish in Peru. The fish is marinated in a lime mixture that breaks down the proteins, meaning it appears to cook without using any heat. This method retains all of the fish's nutrients and health benefits. This makes a great starter if you're cooking for friends, too.

SEA BASS CEVICHE

3 very fresh sea bass fillets, skinned

1 red onion, peeled and finely diced

1 green chilli, deseeded and finely diced

1 yellow pepper, deseeded and finely diced

2 tbsp jalapeño Tabasco (green)

1 tbsp light olive oil

juice of 2 limes

salt, to taste

a few small basil leaves

Slice the fillets of sea bass into wafer-thin pieces and place them in a bowl.

Add the red onion, chilli and pepper to the bowl then stir in the Tabasco, oil, lime juice and salt. Mix well and leave to stand for 2–3 minutes.

Divide the fish and vegetables between 2 bowls and garnish with the basil leaves to serve.

// NUTRITION PER SERVING: CALORIES 361 / FAT 17G / CARBS 17G / PROTEIN 35G

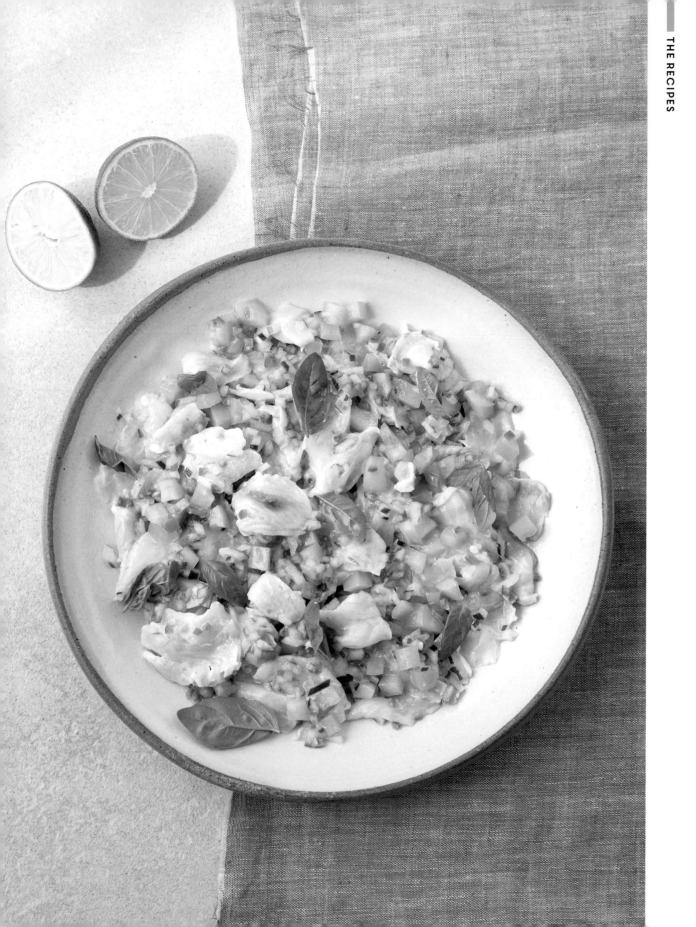

This proves salads don't need to be dull. **A** veggie, grains and feta combo, it is perfect for a workday lunch.

GREEK COUSCOUS SALAD

600ml chicken stock

2 tbsp olive oil

½ tsp sea salt

200g dry couscous

½ tsp dried basil

½ tsp dried dill

1 tsp garlic powder

pinch dried marjoram

65g feta

2 large tomatoes, diced

1 medium cucumber, diced

130g Kalamata olives, pitted

drizzle balsamic vinegar

Pour the stock into a large saucepan and bring to the boil over a medium heat.

Once the stock is boiling, turn down the heat, then stir in 1 teaspoon of the olive oil and the salt and mix well.

Add the dry couscous and simmer for 1–2 minutes before removing from the heat. Leave the couscous to sit for 5–6 minutes, until most of the liquid has been absorbed.

Fluff up the couscous with a fork, then stir in the basil, dill, garlic powder and marjoram and mix very well. Stir through the remaining olive oil until the couscous is coated.

Add most of the feta and all of the tomatoes, cucumber and olives and stir until fully mixed together.

Top with the remaining feta and drizzle with balsamic to serve.

// NUTRITION PER SERVING: CALORIES 503 / FAT 15G / CARBS 73G / PROTEIN 16G

SERVES 2

Feel like chicken tonight? Here's a lighter way to tuck in. It travels well, too, so pack it up as a healthy lunch. It's best if you marinate the chicken in advance - but don't worry if you want this instantly, the meal works even if you don't.

PROTEIN POWERHOUSE CHICKEN SALAD

2 free-range skinless chicken breasts, cut into 2cm strips

1 tbsp olive oil

1 tbsp ground cumin

½ tbsp ground coriander

½ tbsp paprika

juice of 2 limes

200g frozen sweetcorn, defrosted

250g cooked quinoa

150g cherry tomatoes, halved

4 spring onions, trimmed and finely sliced

2 red chillies, deseeded and diced

a handful of fresh coriander leaves, roughly chopped

1 avocado, peeled, destoned and diced

sea salt and freshly ground black pepper

Place the chicken, oil, cumin, ground coriander and paprika in a bowl, and squeeze over half a lime. Mix so the chicken has a good coating of the oil and spices. Leave to marinate for 2 hours, if possible.

Place a large frying pan over a high heat and fry the chicken for 10 minutes, or until cooked through. Season with salt and pepper. Take the chicken out of the pan and set aside.

Using the same pan, cook the sweetcorn until it begins to colour.

Take the pan off the heat and add the quinoa, tomatoes, spring onions, chilli, fresh coriander and the remaining lime juice. Mix everything together until it has a good covering.

Transfer to 2 plates, top with the diced avocado and chicken and serve.

// NUTRITION PER SERVING: CALORIES 681 / FAT 33G / CARBS 65G / PROTEIN 41G

SERVES 4

If you get the ripest tomatoes, this dish can look like glistening gems in a bowl. I recommend using a variety of tomatoes, like green zebra, golden sunrise, big red and mixed cherry tomatoes. Pomegranate molasses (made by reducing down pomegranate juice to make a thick, intense syrup) is one of my favourite ingredients. In the dressing here, it gives a more complex flavour than you'd get with lemon juice or vinegar, and perfectly complements the tomatoes.

TOMATO, HERB & FETA SALAD WITH POMEGRANATE DRESSING

a bunch of fresh flat-leaf parsley leaves
30g fresh basil leaves
500g tomatoes (you want a good variation of size and colour)
2 small red onions, peeled and sliced very thin
150g feta
4 tbsp pomegranate seeds

FOR THE DRESSING
2 tbsp white balsamic vinegar
2 tbsp pomegranate molasses
1 garlic clove, crushed
pepper, to taste
3 tbsp extra-virgin olive oil
lemon juice, to taste

To make the dressing, measure the balsamic vinegar, pomegranate molasses and crushed garlic into a small bowl.

Season with pepper. Whisk, then add the oil, taste for seasoning and add the lemon juice.

To make the salad, separate some of the best-shaped parsley and basil leaves and leave them whole, then chop the rest.

Cut the tomatoes into slices, or in half if they're small. Put them all into a serving dish and top with the chopped parsley, chopped basil and red onions.

Drizzle with the dressing.

Crumble the feta over the top of the salad and toss gently, being careful not to break up the feta too much.

Sprinkle with the pomegranate seeds and reserved whole parsley and basil leaves and serve.

// NUTRITION PER SERVING: CALORIES 278 / FAT 21G / CARBS 17G / PROTEIN 7G

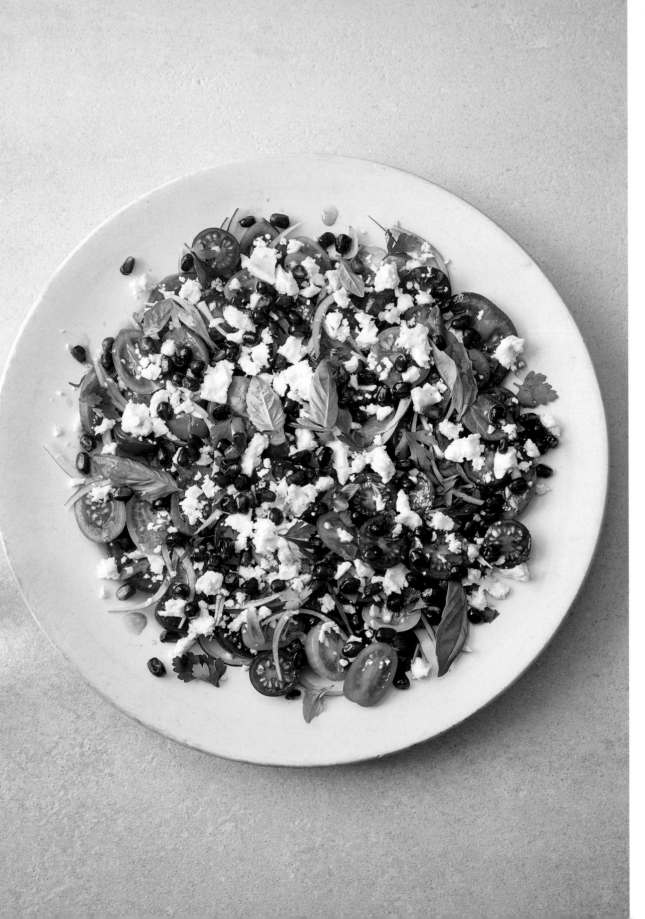

SERVES 8

Quinoa is often hailed as a superfood because it's one of the few plant foods that contain all the amino acids. This is quick to make and a light, delicious vegan salad. Great for a summer barbecue if you have friends over. And just in case you don't know, it's pronounced 'keen-wah'...

SUPERGREEN QUINOA SALAD

1kg quinoa

500g frozen edamame beans

400g frozen peas

4 spring onions, trimmed and
   sliced

3 cucumbers, seeded and diced

4 ripe avocados, peeled, destoned
   and sliced

juice of 4 lemons and zest of 2

60g fresh flat-leaf parsley,
   chopped

60g fresh mint, chopped

3 tbsp olive oil

sea salt and freshly ground black
   pepper

Cook the quinoa following the instructions on the packet. Leave to cool. You can do this in advance and keep it in the fridge.

Steam the edamame beans and peas for 2–3 minutes then leave to cool.

When you're ready to mix the salad, tip the quinoa into a large bowl, add the peas, edamame, spring onions, cucumber, avocado, lemon zest and chopped parsley and mint.

Add the lemon juice and olive oil and check the seasoning. Mix together well and serve.

// NUTRITION PER SERVING: CALORIES 542 / FAT 26G / CARBS 63G / PROTEIN 21G

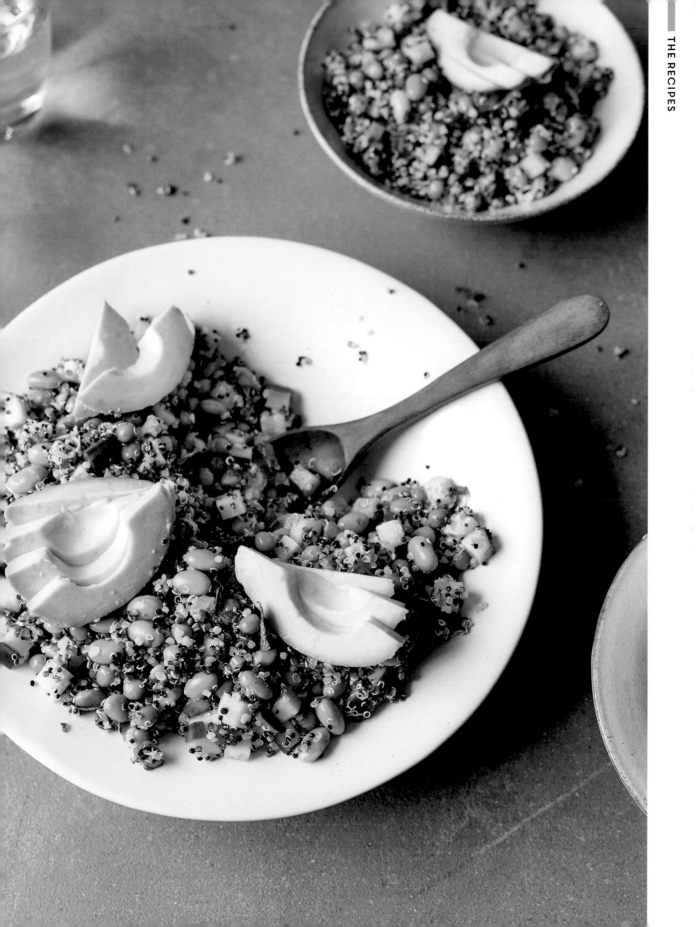

A Japanese delicacy, the word sashimi means 'pierced body'. You need to be very careful to buy the right kind of salmon for this - salmon used for sashimi has been frozen at a very low temperature. Make sure you go to a reputable fishmonger and ask for sashimi-grade salmon. And be sure to buy the pink peppercorns, as this recipe will not work with regular black peppercorns.

SALMON SASHIMI

500g salmon fillet (best quality you can afford and as fresh as possible)

40g red onion, peeled and very finely chopped

2 tbsp pomegranate seeds

1 tbsp pink peppercorns

1 lemon

snipped chives and chopped parsley, to garnish

drizzle olive oil

sea salt

Slice the salmon into 5mm slices or thinner if you can – the thinner the salmon the better it will taste.

Lay the slices on a serving plate and sprinkle over the onion, pomegranate seeds and peppercorns.

Squeeze the lemon over the salmon and garnish with the chives and parsley. Drizzle with olive oil and season with a pinch of sea salt.

// NUTRITION PER SERVING: CALORIES 253 / FAT 14G / CARBS 3G / PROTEIN 27G

SERVES 2

A super simple yet impressive dish of rare steak, Parmesan and rocket: the perfect quick supper after a hard day at work. Look for heritage or beef tomatoes with a rich, full flavour and a hunk of Parmigiano Reggiano, the king of cheeses. The Italians usually make this with sirloin, but I recommend rump. If you can afford to go organic and grass-fed, do.

BEEF TAGLIATA

2 x 200g rump steaks
2 tbsp olive oil
10 heritage tomatoes, cut into
    segments
60g wild rocket
20ml balsamic vinegar
1 tbsp extra-virgin olive oil
40g Parmesan, shaved (best to
    use Parmigiano Reggiano)
sea salt and freshly ground
    black pepper

Trim the fat off the steaks and season both sides generously with salt and pepper.

Place a griddle pan over a high heat and add the olive oil.

Place the steaks in the hot pan and sear for 2 minutes on each side for a rare steak. (If you prefer a medium steak, cook for another minute each side.)

Remove the steaks from the pan and set aside, covered with foil, to rest.

Add the tomatoes to the same pan and cook for 1 minute, until they have coloured and softened slightly.

Place the rocket in a large bowl and dress with the balsamic vinegar and extra-virgin olive oil. Mix with your hands to make sure each leaf is coated lightly.

Cut the steaks into thin slices about 1cm thick.

Arrange the tomatoes on two plates, then top with the rocket and finally the steak.

Finish with Parmesan shavings and serve.

// NUTRITION PER SERVING: CALORIES 610 / FAT 50G / CARBS 20G / PROTEIN 20G

Duck is a rich meat, loaded with protein. I always feel that as meats go, it gets a bad rap. People think duck's unhealthy - maybe they associate it with overdosing on Chinese takeaway. Duck breasts are as lean as chicken or turkey, and contain more iron per serving than most other poultry. Don't duck the duck!

HOISIN & GINGER DUCK SALAD

2 duck breasts

2 pinches Chinese five spice powder

2–3 cucumbers, sliced into fine ribbons with a peeler

1 large baby gem lettuce, finely sliced

1 large carrot, peeled then flesh peeled into ribbons

2 tbsp finely snipped fresh chives

1 heaped tsp minced ginger

juice of 1 lime

1 tbsp water

2 tsp Hoisin sauce

16 cashew nuts, roughly chopped

sea salt and freshly ground black pepper

Season the duck breasts with salt, pepper and a pinch of Chinese five spice.

Place a frying pan over a medium heat and lay the breasts skin side down. Allow the fat to render out of the skin gently for about 10 minutes, then turn and cook the breasts for a further 3 minutes on the flesh side (this will make the duck medium rare – cook it for slightly longer if you prefer).

Remove from the heat and leave to rest.

Meanwhile, combine the cucumber, baby gem, carrot and chives together in a bowl.

In a separate bowl, mix together the ginger, lime juice, water, Hoisin and a pinch of Chinese five spice to make a dressing.

Pour the dressing over the salad and toss to coat.

Slice the duck breast and place on top of the salad. Scatter over the cashews and serve.

// NUTRITION PER SERVING: CALORIES 368 / FAT 22G / CARBS 24G / PROTEIN 22G

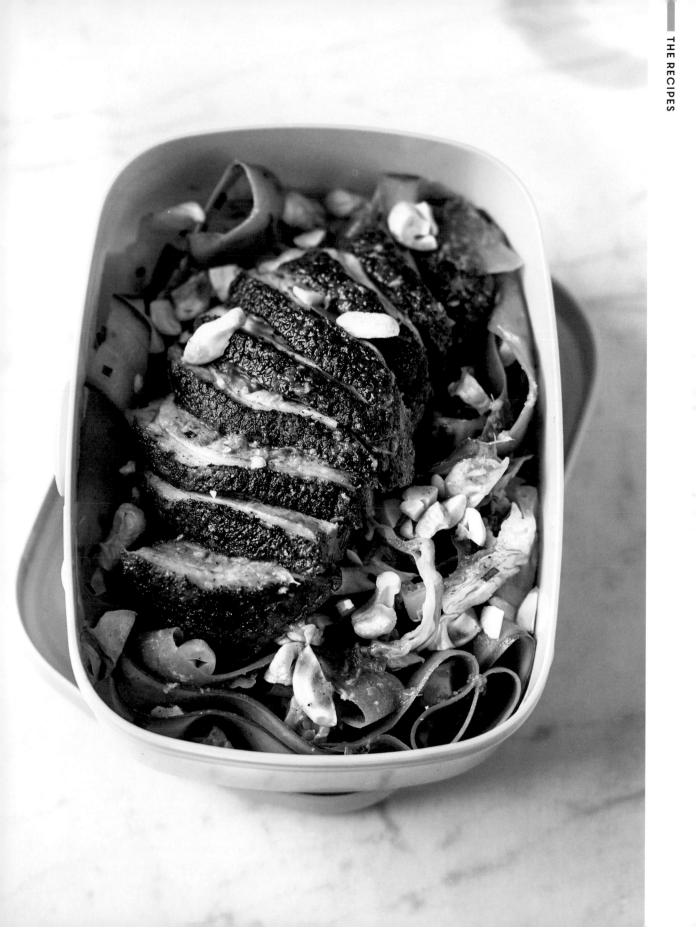

SERVES 2

From a nutrition point of view, you'll struggle to find a more perfect meal than this: the cod is a good source of omega-3 fats and vitamin B12 and the Puy lentils fill you up. But, frankly, you'll forget all that when it goes in your mouth, because you'll be blown away by the taste.

COD IN A BAG

2 x 220g cod fillets (skin on)

1 x 250g ready-to-eat Puy lentils

300g vine tomatoes, quartered

sea salt and freshly ground black
  pepper

FOR THE SAUCE

60g fresh parsley

15g fresh mint

15g fresh basil

1 tbsp capers

½ round shallot, peeled and
  roughly chopped

juice of ½ lemon

1 garlic clove, peeled and finely
  chopped

2 tbsp olive oil

1 tbsp Dijon mustard

FOR THE SALAD

1 bulb fennel, trimmed and thinly
  sliced

zest of ½ lemon

pinch of sea salt

1 tbsp extra-virgin olive oil

2 tsp white wine vinegar

Preheat the oven to 220°C/Fan 200°C and prepare 2 sheets of baking paper, each large enough to wrap a fillet. Take the cod from the fridge to remove the chill and season with salt and pepper.

First make the sauce by placing the parsley, mint, basil, capers, shallot, lemon juice, garlic, olive oil and mustard in a blender and whizzing until the mixture is a smooth paste.

In a bowl, combine the lentils and tomatoes with 4 tablespoons of the sauce and mix well.

Spoon a bed of lentils on to each piece of baking paper and place the fish on top.

Wrap each fillet in the baking paper, securing it with kitchen string, and place both parcels on a baking tray. Bake in the hot oven for 18 minutes.

While the cod is baking, place the fennel in a large bowl. Add the lemon zest, salt, extra-virgin olive oil and vinegar and mix well to ensure each slice of fennel is coated.

Remove the fish from the oven and serve with a generous spoonful of salad and a drizzle of the remaining sauce.

// NUTRITION PER SERVING: CALORIES 423 / FAT 21G / CARBS 29G / PROTEIN 31G

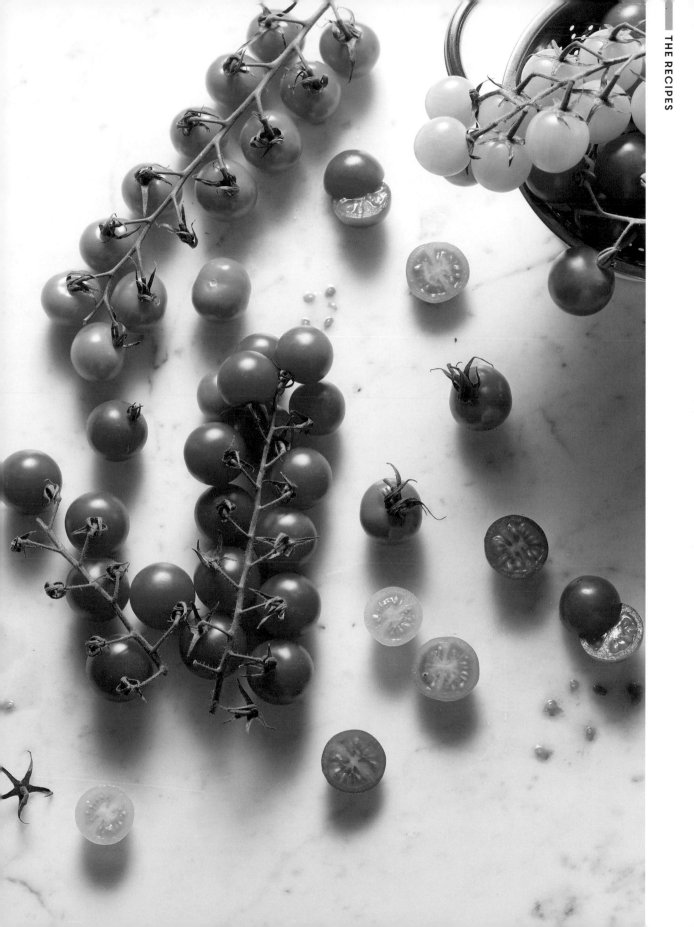

SERVES 2

Packed with vibrant flavours, this will quickly become a new favourite - especially on a wintry day when you want a hot lunch. Cabbage deserves a much better press. It's almost nature's acne remedy, helping dry up oily skin and thus reducing potential breakouts.

SEARED BEEF WITH BURNT CABBAGE

400g sirloin steak, cut into 2cm-long strips

1 tbsp soy sauce

1 tbsp minced ginger

1 tbsp sunflower oil, plus extra for coating

½ white cabbage, chopped into 2–3cm chunks

1 red pepper, finely sliced (julienne)

2 generous handfuls of beansprouts

a handful of fresh coriander leaves, roughly chopped

1 tbsp sesame seeds

Combine the steak with the soy sauce and ginger in a bowl. Leave to marinate for 20 minutes.

Lightly coat a frying pan with sunflower oil and place over a high heat.

When hot, add the steak and sear until cooked to your satisfaction.

Place another frying pan (ideally cast iron) over a high heat until it is almost smoking. Add 1 tablespoon of sunflower oil to the pan, then the cabbage. Let the cabbage catch – only stir it 2–3 times over the course of 4–5 minutes. Allow it to burn!

Add the red pepper to the pan and cook for 1 minute.

Add the beansprouts and cook for a further minute.

Remove from the heat and divide evenly between 2 plates.

Serve with the beef resting on top then sprinkle each plate with the fresh coriander and sesame seeds.

// NUTRITION PER SERVING: CALORIES 585 / FAT 36G / CARBS 23G / PROTEIN 47G

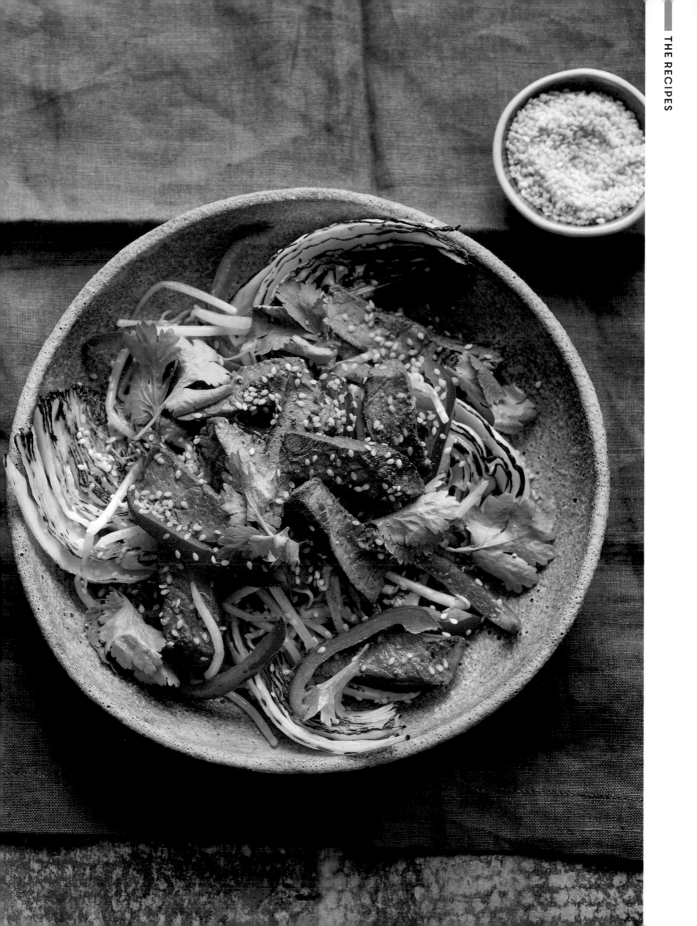

SERVES 2

There's something wonderful about the tartness of grapefruit combined with the creaminess of avocado. This is best enjoyed in the winter and spring when grapefruit is in season.

AVOCADO & GRAPEFRUIT SALAD

1 pink grapefruit, segmented with juice reserved

heaped tsp Dijon mustard

3 tbsp olive oil

1½ tbsp sherry vinegar

1 fennel, finely sliced with a mandolin

200g cooked quinoa

handful of roughly chopped mint leaves

1 avocado, cut into chunks

sea salt and freshly ground black pepper

Whisk together the reserved grapefruit juice, Dijon mustard, olive oil and sherry vinegar in a bowl to form the dressing.

Combine sliced fennel, quinoa and mint with half of the dressing and season to taste.

Divide between 2 plates and add half the avocado and half the grapefruit segments to each plate. Drizzle with the remaining dressing to taste and serve.

// NUTRITION PER SERVING: CALORIES 144 / FAT 14G / CARBS 6G / PROTEIN 3G

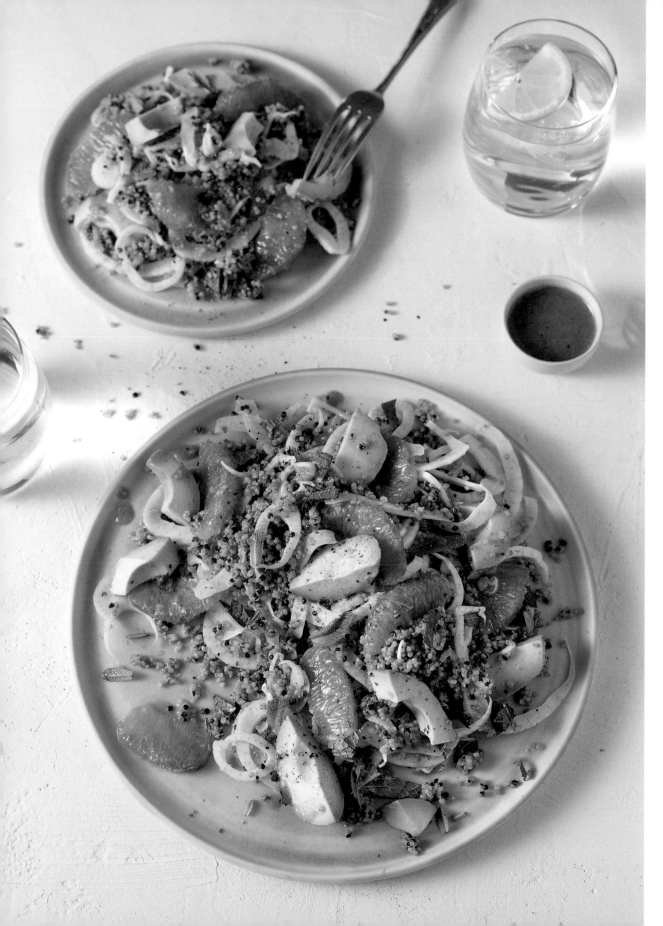

SERVES 2

This is an excellent way to cook aubergine with an oriental twist. This dish goes really well with salmon or steamed tenderstem broccoli dressed with a little cold-pressed toasted sesame oil.

WHITE MISO ROASTED AUBERGINE

1 large aubergine, trimmed
  and chopped into 3cm chunks

2 tbsp coconut oil

2 tbsp white miso

1 tbsp mirin

2 spring onions, trimmed
  and sliced lengthways

a small bunch of fresh
  coriander leaves

1 tsp sesame seeds

Preheat the oven to 160°C/Fan 140°C.

Place the aubergine in a bowl and add the coconut oil.

Tip on to a baking tray and roast in the oven for 15 minutes, then turn the pieces over and roast for a further 15 minutes, until golden brown.

Meanwhile, mix the white miso and mirin together in a small bowl.

Remove the aubergine from the oven and pour the mixture over the top. Return to the oven and roast for another 20 minutes, until the liquid starts to caramelise.

Remove from the oven, top with the spring onions, coriander and sesame seeds and serve.

// NUTRITION PER SERVING: CALORIES 127 / FAT 2G / CARBS 24G / PROTEIN 5G

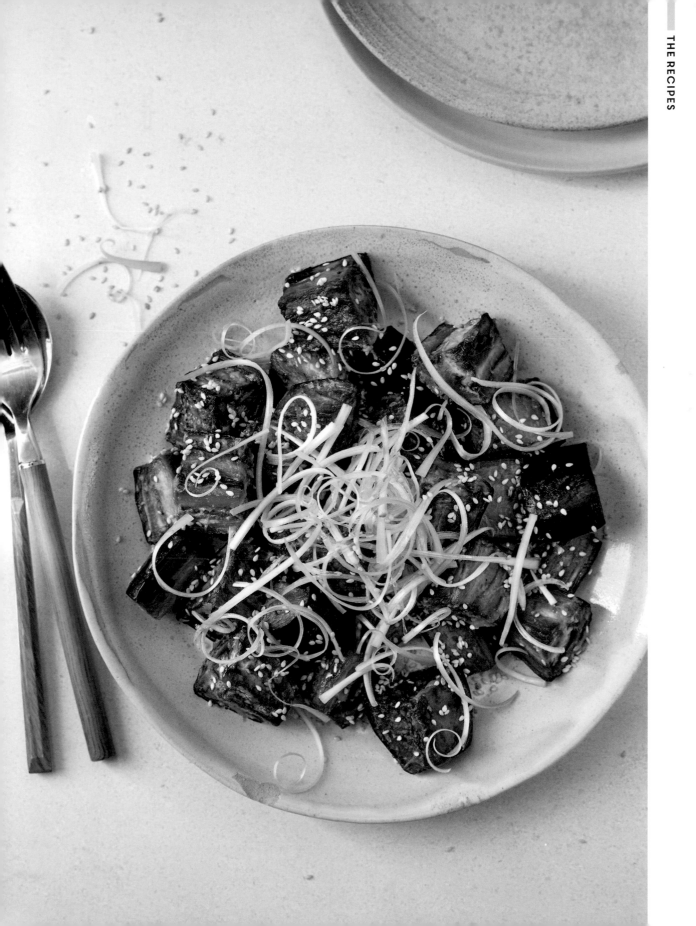

SERVES 4

An everyday classic. I'm a big fan of the spud - the humble potato is fat-free and unfairly maligned by the fitness community.

LAMB & MASH

1kg Maris Piper potatoes, peeled and cut into quarters

1 tbsp coconut oil

2 whole ultra-trimmed racks of lamb

3 garlic cloves, peeled and crushed

400g cherry vine tomatoes

50g butter

50ml milk

sea salt and freshly ground black pepper

Put the potatoes into a large saucepan and cover with water. Place over a high heat and bring to the boil. Reduce the heat to medium-low, cover loosely and simmer gently for 15–20 minutes, or until the potatoes break apart easily when pierced with a fork.

Meanwhile, put the oil in a frying pan over a high heat. Cut each rack evenly into single chops. Season the chops with salt and pepper, then add to the pan with the crushed garlic. Cook for 2–3 minutes on each side, or until brown.

Remove the lamb and garlic from the pan and set aside to rest. Using the same pan over a medium heat, cook the cherry tomatoes until they begin to split.

Meanwhile, drain the potatoes well and return them to the saucepan. Place over a low heat and shake gently for 1–2 minutes to get rid of any excess moisture.

Mash the potatoes until no lumps remain. Season with salt and pepper and continue mashing, gradually adding the butter and milk to make the potatoes smooth and creamy.

Divide the mash, chops and tomatoes between 4 plates and serve.

// NUTRITION PER SERVING: CALORIES 345 / FAT 15G / CARBS 18G / PROTEIN 32G

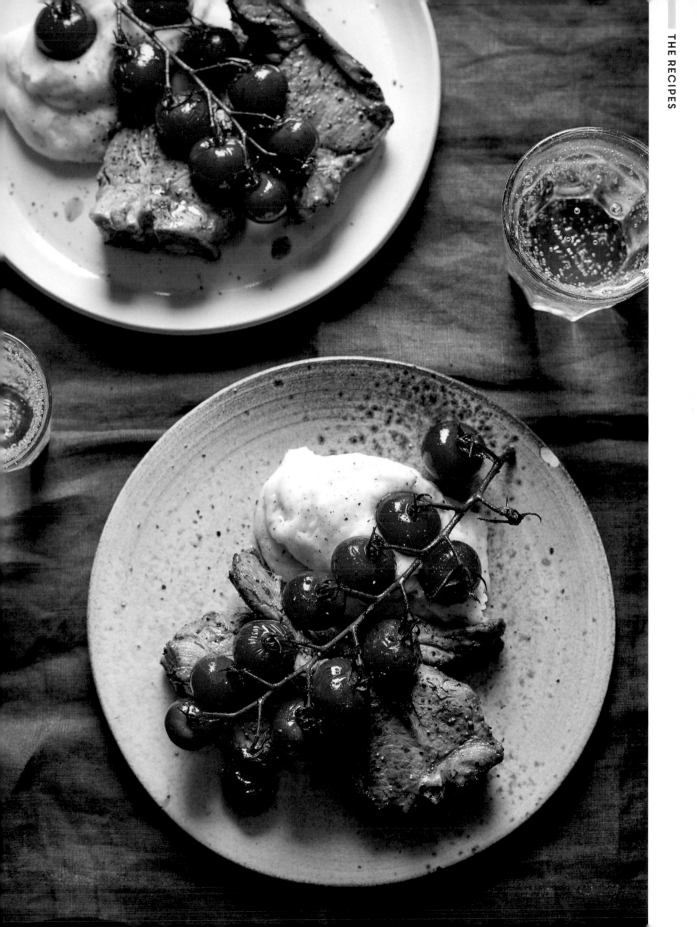

A warming, spicy meal to brighten any cold, wintry day. This is also a great way to eat cauliflower - a very underrated vegetable.

CAULIFLOWER & RED LENTIL CURRY WITH CUCUMBER RAITA

200g dried red lentils

1 medium cauliflower, broken into small florets

1 tbsp ghee or coconut oil

1 red onion, peeled and finely sliced

2 garlic cloves, peeled and crushed

2 tsp curry powder

2 tsp turmeric

2 tsp cumin seeds

1 tsp dried chilli flakes

250g baby spinach leaves, washed

coconut shavings or almonds, to garnish

sea salt and freshly ground black pepper

FOR THE CUCUMBER
& MINT RAITA

2 heaped tbsp coconut yoghurt

¼ cucumber, deseeded and diced (no need to peel)

a handful of fresh mint leaves, finely chopped

To make the raita, mix all the ingredients together in a small bowl and refrigerate.

Rinse and drain the red lentils and place in a large saucepan. Cover with water and bring to the boil. Reduce the heat and simmer gently for 20–25 minutes, until cooked through.

Lightly steam the cauliflower or boil in a large pan of water for a couple of minutes. Drain and set aside.

Place the ghee or coconut oil in a separate large saucepan over a medium heat and add the onion. Cook gently for 8 minutes, until soft, then add the garlic, curry powder, turmeric, cumin seeds and chilli flakes. Season, then cook for another couple of minutes.

Add the cauliflower and stir to coat in the spice mixture.

Finally add the cooked lentils.

Stir everything together well to combine, then add the spinach to wilt softly.

Garnish with coconut shavings or almonds, if using, and serve with steamed vegetables.

// NUTRITION PER SERVING: CALORIES 210 / FAT 8G / CARBS 34G / PROTEIN 11G

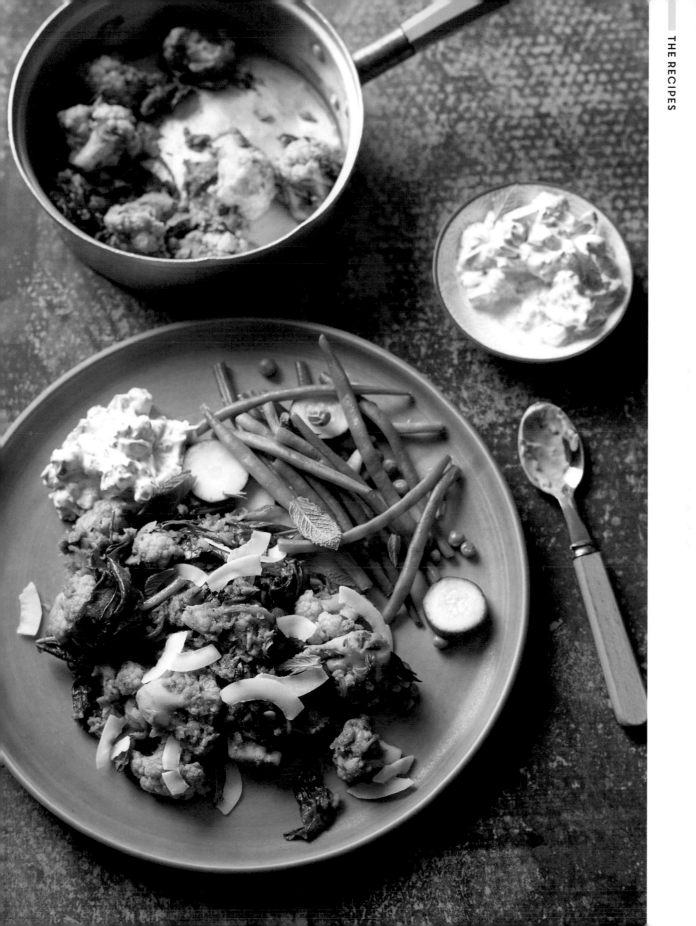

SERVES 2

Who doesn't love a fish pie? This is my twist on an old classic. It's the kind of recipe where you should find you have most of the ingredients in the cupboard already. It can be eaten hot or cold.

SALMON & QUINOA PIE

1 tsp coconut oil

40g quinoa

2 tsp olive oil

1 small onion, peeled and finely chopped

1 garlic clove, peeled and finely chopped

125g butternut squash, peeled and grated

125g broccoli, florets finely chopped

1 x 170g tin wild red Alaskan salmon, skinless and boneless, drained

2 medium free-range eggs, beaten

¼ tsp dried oregano

Preheat the oven to 180°C/Fan 160°C and lightly brush 2 individual pie dishes with a little coconut oil.

Put the quinoa into a sieve and rinse with cold water.

Tip the quinoa into a small saucepan, add 125ml water and bring to the boil. Reduce the heat and simmer gently for 10 minutes, until the water is absorbed.

Meanwhile, heat the oil in a small frying pan over a medium to low heat. Cook the onion and garlic for 8–10 minutes until softened. Remove from the heat and tip into a medium bowl.

Place the squash and broccoli in the bowl with the onion, then add the cooked quinoa, salmon, eggs and oregano. Give everything a thorough mix, breaking up the salmon into big flakes.

Divide between the prepared pie dishes, pressing down a little, and bake in the oven for 25 minutes, until set.

Serve with wilted spinach or a tomato salad.

// NUTRITION PER SERVING: CALORIES 308 / FAT 14G / CARBS 24G / PROTEIN 21G

SERVES 4

A quick Asian-inspired take on a winning combination: salmon and asparagus. And even better, there's very little washing up!

WRAPPED SALMON

225g asparagus, trimmed and
  halved lengthwise
zest and juice of 1 lemon
4 x 150g skinless wild salmon
  fillets
225g shiitake mushrooms, thinly
  sliced
4 spring onions, trimmed and
  thinly sliced
4 tbsp water
sea salt and freshly ground black
  pepper

Preheat the oven to 220°C/Fan 200°C and cut 4 x 45cm pieces of baking paper.

Create 4 x 10cm beds of asparagus spears on each piece of baking paper. Grate a little lemon zest over each pile and season with salt and pepper.

Place a single salmon fillet on top of each bed of spears.

Divide the mushrooms and spring onions evenly between the fillets and place on top.

Add 1 tablespoon of water to each fillet and wrap them up, sealing everything in.

Place all 4 parcels on a baking tray and bake in the oven for 12 minutes. (If you want it well done, bake for 16 minutes.)

Open the parcel at the table and squeeze over some lemon juice to serve.

SERVES 2

Gram for gram, liver is probably more nutritious than any other food - it is loaded with a large spectrum of vitamins, minerals, proteins and fats. Be brave and try it! It will make an interesting change to your standard meal plan.

CALF LIVER WITH CAPERS, CELERIAC & SPINACH

1 celeriac (600g), peeled and cut into 1.5cm dice

3 tsp sunflower oil

1 sprig of thyme, leaves picked

200g baby leaf spinach

2 x 100g slices calf liver

1 tbsp capers

juice of 1 lemon

150ml reduced chicken stock

Dijon mustard, to serve

sea salt and freshly ground black pepper

Preheat the oven to 180°C/Fan 160°C and place a large baking tray in the oven to heat up.

Place the celeriac in a bowl with 1 teaspoon of the sunflower oil, some salt, pepper and the thyme leaves. Use your hands to make sure everything is coated in the herb oil.

Tip on to the hot baking tray and cook in the oven for 20–25 minutes, turning once.

Meanwhile, wash the spinach and place it in a pan over a low heat. Cook for 1–2 minutes, stirring so it doesn't catch. Season, then set aside to keep warm.

Place a non-stick frying pan over a high heat. Rub 1 teaspoon of sunflower oil into each slice of liver and place them in the hot pan to cook for 1–2 minutes on each side. (Cook for longer if you prefer well-done meat.)

Remove from the pan and leave to rest.

Reduce the heat to medium-low and add the capers. Season with pepper and cook for 20 seconds. Add the lemon juice, followed by the chicken stock. It will quickly reduce by half.

Divide the celeriac, spinach and liver between two plates then spoon the sauce over the liver, add the Dijon mustard and serve.

// NUTRITION PER SERVING: CALORIES 184 / FAT 11G / CARBS 12G / PROTEIN 11G

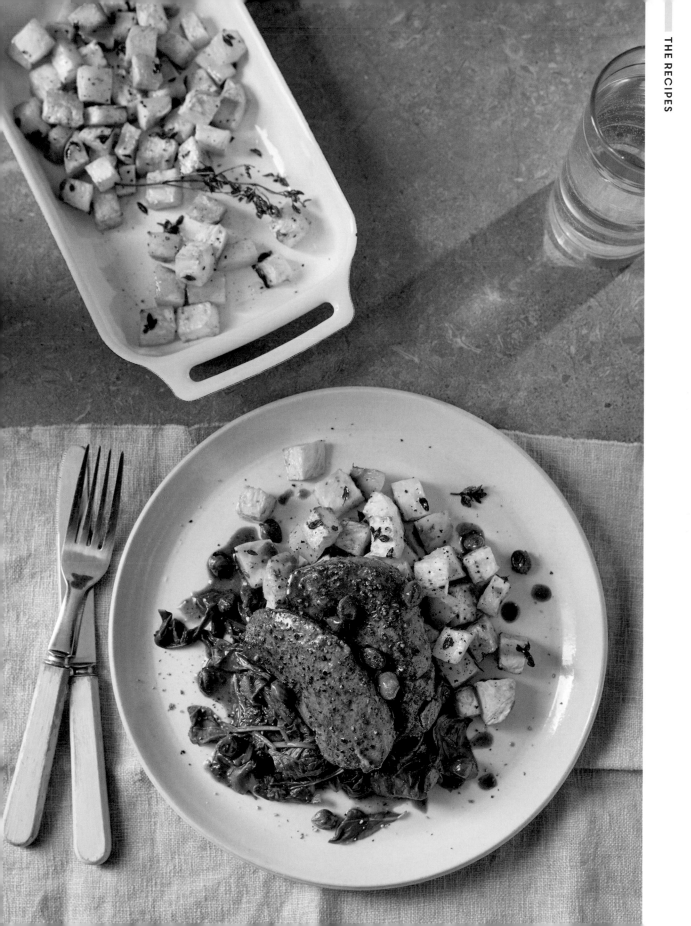

SERVES 2

This is a cheeky name, as there's actually no rice in this dish. What you're really doing is substituting cauliflower for rice to make a dinner that's so delicious, you wouldn't guess that it was also ultra-virtuous.

FRIED CAULIFLOWER RICE

2 medium free-range eggs

1 tsp sesame oil

1 medium cauliflower (approx. 400g), leaves removed and florets roughly chopped into big chunks

1 tbsp groundnut oil

2 spring onions, trimmed and finely chopped

60g frozen mixed vegetables

3 garlic cloves, peeled and minced

3 tbsp tamari (Japanese gluten-free soy sauce)

a small handful of fresh coriander leaves, roughly chopped

a large pinch of sea salt and freshly ground black pepper

Crack the eggs into a bowl and add 1 teaspoon of the sesame oil. Whisk together and set aside.

Grate the cauliflower in a food processor or with a box grater.

Place the groundnut oil in a wok or large non-stick frying pan over a high heat. Add the cauliflower, spring onions and frozen mixed vegetables and stir-fry for 3–4 minutes, until the cauliflower is just beginning to become tender.

Add the garlic and season with salt and pepper. Continue to stir-fry for 30 seconds or so, until the garlic is fragrant but not burnt.

Push the mixture around the sides of the wok to create an opening in the middle and add the beaten eggs. Scramble the eggs, then toss through the mixture to combine.

Drizzle with tamari and mix again.

Serve piping hot, finished with fresh coriander.

// NUTRITION PER SERVING: CALORIES 332 / FAT 19G / CARBS 33G / PROTEIN 11G

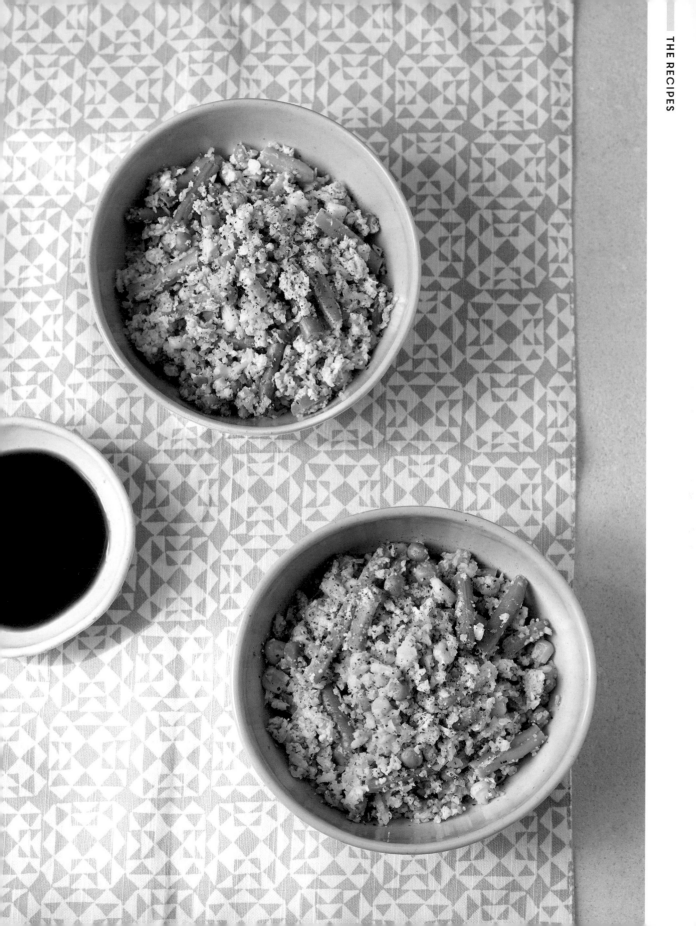

Turkey shouldn't just be for Christmas. It is a fantastic lean meat. And who doesn't love chilli?

TURKEY CHILLI

1 tsp olive oil

1 large onion, peeled and chopped

1 tsp sea salt

2 garlic cloves, peeled and minced

½ tbsp hot chilli flakes

1 tsp ground cinnamon

2 tbsp tomato purée

450g turkey mince

2 x 400g tins chopped tomatoes

1 tsp balsamic vinegar

250g frozen sweetcorn

1 x 400g tin black beans, drained and rinsed

100g mature Cheddar, grated

a handful of fresh coriander leaves, roughly chopped

freshly ground black pepper

Place a large, non-stick frying pan over a medium heat. Add the olive oil, onion and salt, cover and cook for about 10 minutes, until softened.

Turn up the heat a little and add the garlic and chilli. After a minute, stir through the cinnamon and tomato purée.

Add the turkey mince, breaking it into small pieces, and brown the meat for about 5 minutes. Season with pepper.

Stir in the chopped tomatoes, balsamic vinegar, sweetcorn and black beans, cover with a lid and continue to cook for 10–15 minutes.

Remove from the heat and pile on to plates.

Garnish with Cheddar and coriander to serve.

// NUTRITION PER SERVING: CALORIES 273 / FAT 12G / CARBS 37G / PROTEIN 12G

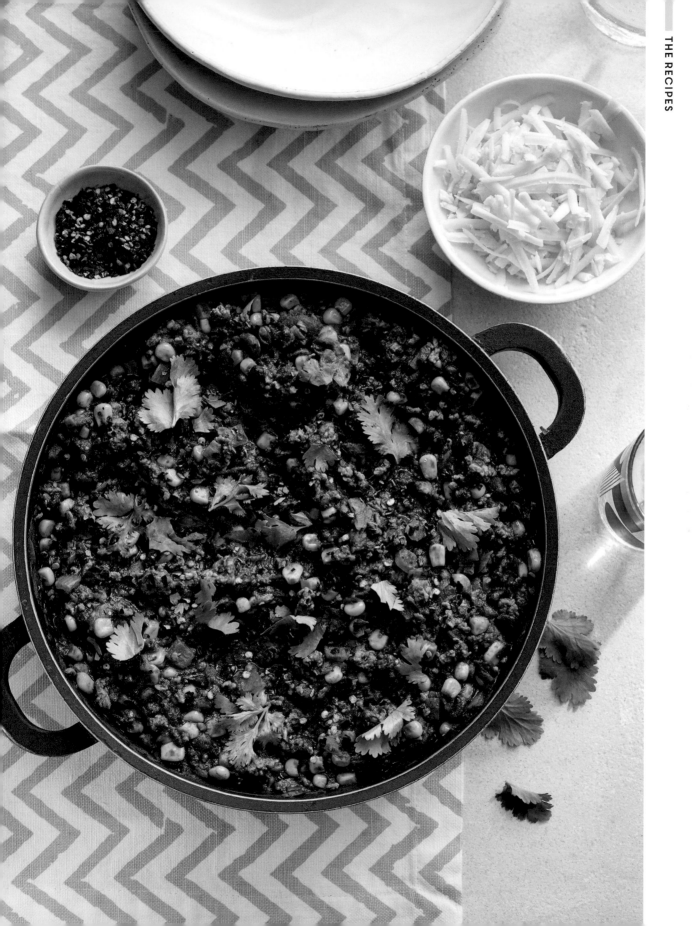

SERVES 2

Chicken is the ultimate comfort food - and it's never better than with garlic. Garlic gets a bad rap. We focus on its breath-ruining properties and overlook the fact that it is a true superfood: it not only keeps vampires away, it is also good for heart health. It is packed with allicin, which has antibacterial, antiviral, antifungal and antioxidant properties. Oh, and if you have garlic breath, nature has a remedy - just chew on some parsley.

GARLIC CHICKEN

450g free-range skinless
    chicken breast
60g red Camargue rice
1 tsp coconut oil
1 large garlic clove, peeled
    and crushed
zest and juice of 1 lemon
650g courgettes, trimmed and
    sliced into half moons
350g peas, frozen or fresh
30g spring onions, trimmed
    and chopped
a small handful of fresh
    parsley leaves
sea salt and freshly ground
    black pepper

Remove the chicken from the fridge and slice into 2cm strips. Season with black pepper.

Put the rice, a generous pinch of salt and 90ml water in a saucepan over a high heat and bring to the boil. Cover with a lid, reduce the heat and simmer for 20 minutes. (If your lid has a steam valve, keep it closed.)

Meanwhile, preheat a heavy-based frying pan over a medium heat and swirl with coconut oil to coat. Add the garlic and lemon zest and cook for 10 seconds.

Add the chicken and a pinch of salt and cook for 10 minutes, stirring occasionally. Transfer to a bowl and set aside.

Using the same pan, add the courgettes and a little more coconut oil if needed. Cook for 5–7 minutes, until slightly golden.

Return the chicken to the pan, along with the peas, spring onions and parsley, and a tablespoon of lemon juice. Check the seasoning.

Remove from the heat and serve. The dish is best served with rice.

// NUTRITION PER SERVING: CALORIES 732 / FAT 24G / CARBS 57G / PROTEIN 77G

SERVES 4

A fragrant slow-cooked Thai dish enriched with coconut cream. The recipe calls for brown rice, but it's even more impressive served with sticky black rice.

CHICKEN, LIME & COCONUT PARCELS

4 x 250g free-range skinless chicken thighs

240g brown rice

2 green chillies, deseeded

2 garlic cloves, peeled

1 tsp minced fresh root ginger

zest and juice of 1 lime

30g fresh coriander, with stalks

1 tbsp cumin seeds

3 tbsp Thai fish sauce

4 tbsp coconut cream

4 banana leaves

15g red chillies, sliced

a handful of fresh Thai basil leaves

pinch of sea salt

You will need a stainless steel or bamboo steamer. Cut 4 pieces of baking paper measuring 30 x 40cm. Remove the chicken from the fridge and pour the rice into a bowl of water to soak.

Place the chillies, garlic, ginger, lime zest and juice, coriander, cumin, fish sauce and coconut cream into a blender and whizz until a smooth paste. Rub this paste over the chicken thighs.

Place one banana leaf on each piece of baking paper and a chicken thigh in the centre of each one. Fold the banana leaf and baking paper tightly around each thigh, securing with kitchen string. Place the parcels in the steamer.

Fill a large pot (one that fits the steamer) halfway with water. Bring to the boil, then reduce to a simmer and carefully place the steamer over the top. Steam the chicken for 1 hour.

Refill the pot with boiling water, then steam for a further hour. Finally, top up the water again and steam for a final 30–45 minutes.

In the last phase of steaming the chicken, bring 500ml of water to the boil in a separate large saucepan. Drain the rice and add to the pan with a generous pinch of salt. Cover with a lid, reduce the heat and leave to simmer for 20 minutes.

Remove from the heat and leave to stand until the chicken is ready.

Serve the fluffy rice with a parcel of chicken and the red chilli and Thai basil on the side.

// NUTRITION PER SERVING: CALORIES 464 / FAT 17G / CARBS 20G / PROTEIN 50G

195

SERVES 4

One of my most cherished possessions at my house is my BBQ. I use it all year round - even in the cold of a London winter! That's the defiant Aussie in me. I love cooking these chicken kebabs on it. They are quick, easy and, best of all, leave very little washing up. Alternatively, you can achieve (almost) the same effect on a griddle pan in your kitchen.

CHICKEN KEBABS

380g free-range skinless and
  boneless chicken thighs,
  cut into 3–4cm pieces
1 green pepper, deseeded and
  cut into chunks
1 red pepper, deseeded and cut
  into chunks
1 tbsp dried oregano
2 garlic cloves, peeled and grated
zest and juice of ½ lemon
½ tbsp extra-virgin olive oil
4 Portobello mushrooms,
  quartered
8 cherry tomatoes
25g feta
sea salt and freshly ground
  black pepper

DRESSING
2 tbsp extra-virgin olive oil
2 tbsp red wine vinegar
2 tbsp water
1 tsp honey
1 garlic clove, peeled and minced
20g Kalamata olives, pitted and
  finely chopped
2 tsp fresh oregano leaves

Place the chicken and the green and red peppers in a large bowl.

Add the oregano, garlic, lemon zest and juice and olive oil and season. Use your hands to make sure everything is well covered.

Cover the bowl and leave in the fridge to marinate for 1 hour. In the meantime, soak 8 wooden skewers (if using) in water and fire up the charcoal BBQ.

Alternate pieces of chicken, green and red pepper and mushroom on to each kebab skewer, finishing each one with a cherry tomato.

Ensure the BBQ or griddle pan is very hot and place the kebabs on to cook for 5 minutes on each side.

Meanwhile, make the dressing by mixing together the olive oil, vinegar, water, honey, garlic, olives and oregano leaves in a small bowl.

Divide the kebabs between the plates, drizzle with the dressing and crumble over the feta.

// NUTRITION PER SERVING: CALORIES 280 / FAT 18G / CARBS 11G / PROTEIN 20G

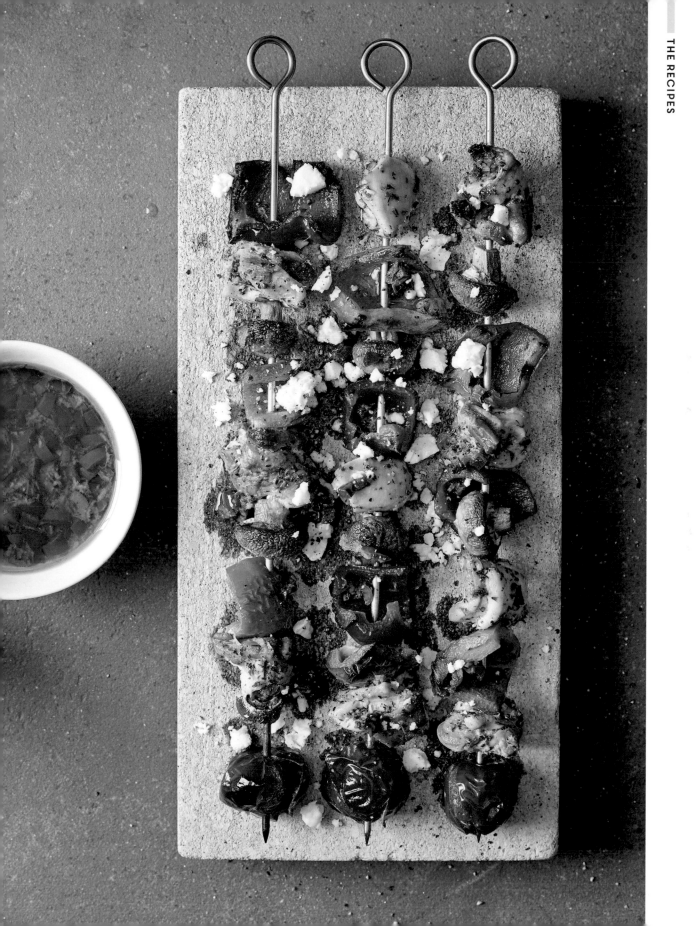

SERVES 4

Cod is an excellent low-calorie protein and is available throughout the year. It's a great substitute for meat and stocks of cod are finally recovering now, too. It is also a good source of omega-3 fatty acids. The recipe only uses the broccoli florets; the stalks can be saved for another day - you could thinly slice them and stir-fry.

BAKED COD WITH BROCCOLI

25ml olive oil

125g wholewheat breadcrumbs

85g full-fat Greek yoghurt

15g Parmesan, grated

5g fresh flat-leaf parsley, finely chopped

5g fresh basil, finely chopped

2 garlic cloves, peeled and finely minced

zest and juice of 1 large lemon

¾ tsp fine sea salt, plus a little extra

½ tsp paprika

¼ tsp freshly ground black pepper, plus a little extra

4 x 150g cod fillets

1 large head broccoli, washed, dried and florets cut into bite-size pieces

1 tsp garlic powder

Preheat the oven to 220°C/Fan 200°C and line two roasting tins with baking paper.

Combine 1 tablespoon of the olive oil with the breadcrumbs in a small bowl and toss them well to coat evenly. Set aside.

Measure the Greek yoghurt, Parmesan, parsley, basil, garlic, lemon zest, sea salt, paprika and freshly ground black pepper into a separate bowl and mix well.

Spoon the yoghurt mixture on to the top of each fillet and spread with the back of a spoon to cover. Press the breadcrumb mixture into the yoghurt on each fillet, then place the fish on one of the prepared roasting tins with the crust side up.

Place all the broccoli florets in a large bowl and dress with the remaining olive oil. Season with the garlic powder and a little salt and pepper. Use your hands to mix everything together to ensure all the florets are evenly coated.

Arrange the broccoli in a single layer on the second roasting tin and place in the oven for 10 minutes.

Turn the broccoli over, then return to the oven, along with the fish, and bake for 12–15 minutes, until each fillet is cooked through.

Serve everything together, finished with a spoonful of lemon juice.

// NUTRITION PER SERVING: CALORIES 250 / FAT 8G / CARBS 18G / PROTEIN 26G

SERVES 4

Sea bass is always an elegant fish - the superstar of
the seas. This is quick and easy, too - a low-effort but
high-reward meal.

SEA BASS IN CRAZY WATER

3 tbsp olive oil

1 white onion, peeled and cut
   into 8 crescents

3 tomatoes, peeled, deseeded
   and cut into small cubes

2 tsp capers (if salted, rinsed)

10 Kalamata olives, pitted

4 basil leaves

4 x 360g sea bass fillets

freshly ground black pepper
   (optional)

Put the olive oil, onion, tomatoes, capers and olives into a
wide frying pan and place over a medium heat. Cook for 15–20
minutes, adding a little water if it starts to catch on the base.
Add the basil leaves and sea bass, skin side down, cover with a
lid and cook for another 8–10 minutes.

Remove from the heat, season with pepper, if liked, and serve.

SERVES 2

A very handsome and impressive dish to serve, though it is easy to make - one for a special guest.

ITALIAN BAKED SEA BASS

1 x 290g jar whole roasted
   peppers, drained and sliced
1 red onion, peeled and sliced
   into very thin wedges
a drizzle of olive oil
1 lemon
4 garlic cloves
2 x 300g sea bass, scaled and
   gutted
15 black olives
25g pine nuts, toasted
a handful of fresh parsley
   leaves, roughly chopped
sea salt and freshly ground
   black pepper

Preheat the oven to 220°C/Fan 200°C.

Toss the peppers and onions in a bowl with the olive oil and season with salt and pepper.

Spread the vegetables in a roasting tin and cook in the oven for 5 minutes.

Cut 3 fat slices of lemon and cut the rest into wedges to serve.

Remove the tin from the oven and add the garlic cloves and fat lemon slices. Place the sea bass on top, brush the fish with a little more oil and season. Roast in the oven for another 15 minutes.

Finally, scatter the olives and pine nuts over the fish and roast for a final 5 minutes, until the fish is just cooked through.

Sprinkle with parsley and serve with a lemon wedge on the side.

// **NUTRITION PER SERVING: CALORIES 498 / FAT 25G / CARBS 16G / PROTEIN 47G**

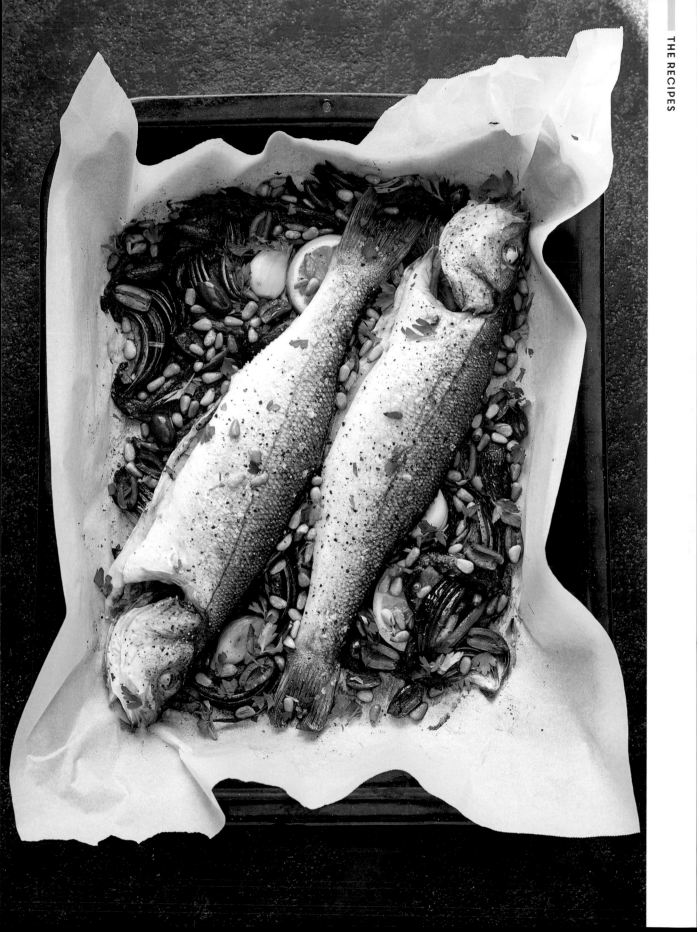

SERVES 2

A light, modern take on a traditional 19th-century Chinese dish - ultra-filling and moreish.

KUNG PAO CHICKEN WITH COURGETTE PASTA

2 medium courgettes (about 225g each), ends trimmed

1 tsp grape seed or canola oil

170g free-range skinless chicken breasts, cut into 2cm pieces

1 tsp sesame oil

2 garlic cloves, peeled and finely chopped

1 tsp ground ginger

½ red pepper, deseeded and cut into 2cm pieces

2 tbsp dry-roasted peanuts, crushed

2 spring onions, trimmed and thinly sliced along the diagonal

sea salt and freshly ground black pepper

CHILLI SAUCE

1½ tbsp reduced salt soy sauce

1 tbsp balsamic vinegar

1 tsp Hoisin sauce

2½ tbsp water

½ tbsp sambal oelek red chilli paste (or more, to taste)

2 tsp honey

2 tsp cornflour

Using a spiralizer with the thickest noodle blade or a mandolin fitted with a julienne blade, cut the courgettes into long spaghetti-like strips. If you are using a spiralizer, use kitchen scissors to cut the strands into pieces about 15–20cm long so they're easier to eat.

To make the chilli sauce, whisk the soy sauce, balsamic, Hoisin, water, red chilli paste, honey and cornflour together in a small bowl. Set aside.

Heat the grape seed or canola oil in a large, deep, non-stick frying pan or wok over a medium to high heat.

Season the chicken with salt and pepper and add to the pan. Cook for 4–5 minutes, until browned and cooked through. Remove from the pan with a slotted spoon and set aside. Reduce the heat to medium and add the sesame oil, garlic and ginger to the pan. Cook for about 30 seconds, until fragrant.

Add the red pepper, then stir in the chilli sauce and bring to the boil. Reduce the heat and simmer for 1–2 minutes, until thickened and bubbling.

Stir in the courgette noodles and cook, stirring, for about 2 minutes, until just tender. If it seems dry, don't worry, the courgettes will release moisture.

Remove from the heat, mix in the chicken and divide between 2 bowls. Top with the peanuts and sliced spring onions and serve.

// NUTRITION PER SERVING: CALORIES 423 / FAT 22G / CARBS 17G / PROTEIN 28G

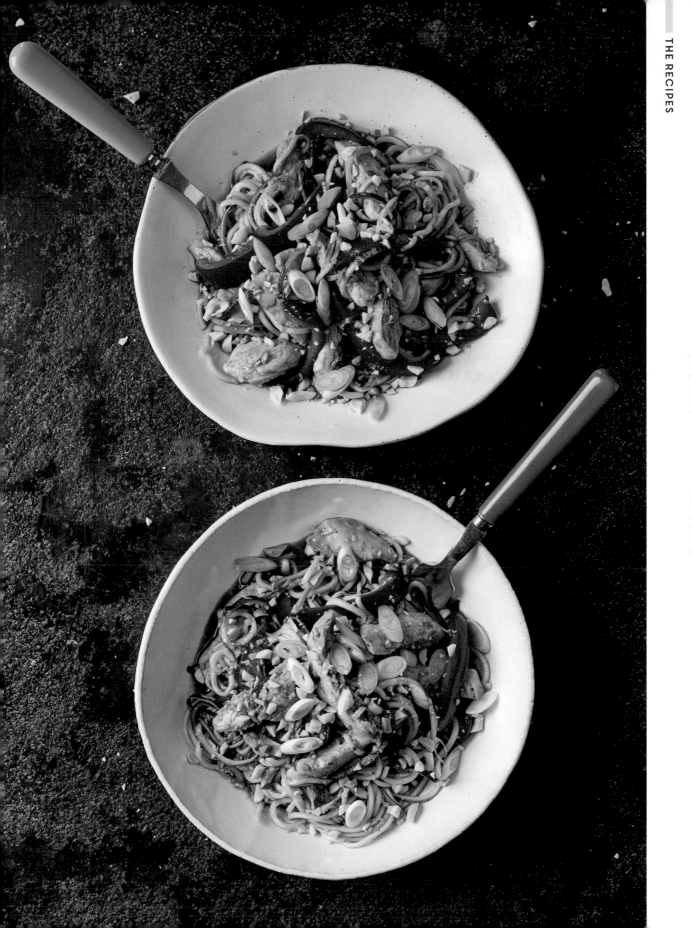

SERVES 2

A good recipe to whip up when friends are coming for dinner: just scale up the ingredients as needed. Choose either soft and delicate lettuce leaves, such as butter lettuce, or crunchy baby gem or chicory.

ASIAN LETTUCE BURRITO

250g turkey mince

½ tbsp groundnut oil

1 small white onion, peeled and diced

2 tbsp Hoisin sauce

½ tbsp soy sauce

½ tbsp rice wine vinegar

1 tsp finely minced fresh root ginger

1 x 225g tin water chestnuts, drained and finely chopped

2 lettuce heads, leaves separated, washed and patted dry

90g spring onions, trimmed and finely chopped

a small handful of fresh mint leaves, finely sliced

2 tsp sesame oil

Remove the turkey mince from the fridge to remove the chill.

Heat the oil in a large frying pan or wok over a medium heat. Add the onion, stirring constantly for 10 minutes, until soft and lightly browned.

Add the turkey mince, breaking it up with a wooden spoon, and fry lightly for a few minutes, until golden brown.

Stir in the Hoisin, soy, vinegar, ginger and water chestnuts and remove from the heat.

Meanwhile, arrange the lettuce leaves on a plate. Spoon some turkey mince into each one and finish with the spring onions, fresh mint and sesame oil.

// NUTRITION PER SERVING: CALORIES 348 / FAT 22G / CARBS 21G / PROTEIN 21G

SERVES 2

An effortlessly easy dinner for two that also makes a
fantastic BBQ. Prepare the chicken and chimichurri sauce
the night before if you have time. Look out for sheep
ricotta, which is more flavoursome than the cows' milk
variety, or you could use goats' curd.

CHICKEN & CHIMICHURRI

2 free-range skinless chicken
 breasts
2 tbsp olive oil
1 tsp paprika
350ml red wine vinegar
1 garlic clove, peeled and
 crushed
1 tsp dried oregano
2 tbsp extra-virgin olive oil
1 tsp finely chopped red
 chilli, deseeded
30g flat-leaf parsley
90g rocket
½ red onion, peeled and diced
30g fresh coriander, leaves only
65g Kalamata olives, pitted
60g ricotta cheese
sea salt and freshly ground
 black pepper

Place the chicken breasts on a chopping board and cover them
with baking paper. Beat each one flat with a meat tenderiser or
rolling pin, until they are about 1.5cm thick.

Combine the olive oil, paprika and a generous pinch of freshly
ground black pepper in a large bowl.

Place the chicken in the bowl and coat with the paprika mixture.
Cover and leave in the fridge overnight, or for at least 20 minutes.

Remove the chicken from the fridge and place a large griddle
pan over a medium to high heat.

When the pan is hot, add the chicken and cook for 4–5 minutes on
each side, until cooked through. Do not be tempted to move the
chicken once it is in the pan or it will lose the char lines. Remove
from the heat, cover with foil and set aside to rest for a few minutes.

Meanwhile, make the chimichurri sauce by combining the
vinegar, garlic, oregano, olive oil, chilli, parsley and a pinch of
salt and pepper in a blender and whizzing until smooth.

In a large bowl, combine the rocket, onion, coriander and
olives. Add the chimichurri sauce and use your hands to mix.
Make sure the leaves are evenly coated.

Cut the chicken into thin slices. Divide the salad between 2 plates
and top with the chicken. Finish by crumbling over a little ricotta.

// NUTRITION PER SERVING: CALORIES 381 / FAT 25G / CARBS 3G / PROTEIN 36G

SERVES 4

Miso paste has an umami quality that pairs perfectly with the fattiness of salmon, while also keeping the fish tender and succulent. Look for tenderstem or purple sprouting broccoli if you can find it, and baby broad beans or even peas make a good alternative to edamame. The salmon is better if prepped the night before.

MISO SALMON WITH BLACK BEAN NOODLES

6 tbsp white miso paste

5 tbsp mirin

5 tbsp soy sauce

2½ tsp minced fresh root ginger

1 tbsp agave nectar

3 tbsp groundnut oil

4 x 150g salmon fillets

680g tenderstem broccoli florets, ends trimmed

680g edamame

340g young carrots, washed and trimmed

400g black bean noodles

a small handful of fresh coriander leaves

juice of 1 lime

1 tbsp sesame seeds, toasted

sea salt and white pepper

In a large bowl, combine the miso, mirin, soy sauce, ginger, agave and 2 tablespoons of the groundnut oil. Add the salmon and coat with the mixture. Cover and place in the fridge to marinate overnight, or for at least 20 minutes.

Preheat the oven to 200°C/Fan 180°C and line a roasting tin with baking paper. Remove the salmon from the fridge.

Place the broccoli, edamame and carrots in a large bowl and dress with the remaining oil. Season with sea salt and white pepper.

Lift the salmon into the roasting tin and arrange the vegetables around the fillets. Roast for 15–20 minutes, until the miso has baked to a rich, golden brown and the salmon is just cooked through. There should still be a little bite to the vegetables.

Meanwhile, bring a large saucepan of water to the boil. Add the noodles, reduce the heat and simmer for 7–8 minutes, or until tender but still retaining their shape. Remove from the heat and strain. Set aside to cool slightly.

Divide the veg between 4 plates, top with the salmon and noodles and finish with a little coriander, a squeeze of lime and a scattering of sesame seeds.

TIP:
Mirin is a Japanese sweet rice wine that makes a dish slightly acidic. You can use rice vinegar, sweet Marsala wine, dry white wine or even dry sherry as substitutes.

// NUTRITION PER SERVING: CALORIES 836 / FAT 30G / CARBS 82G / PROTEIN 60G

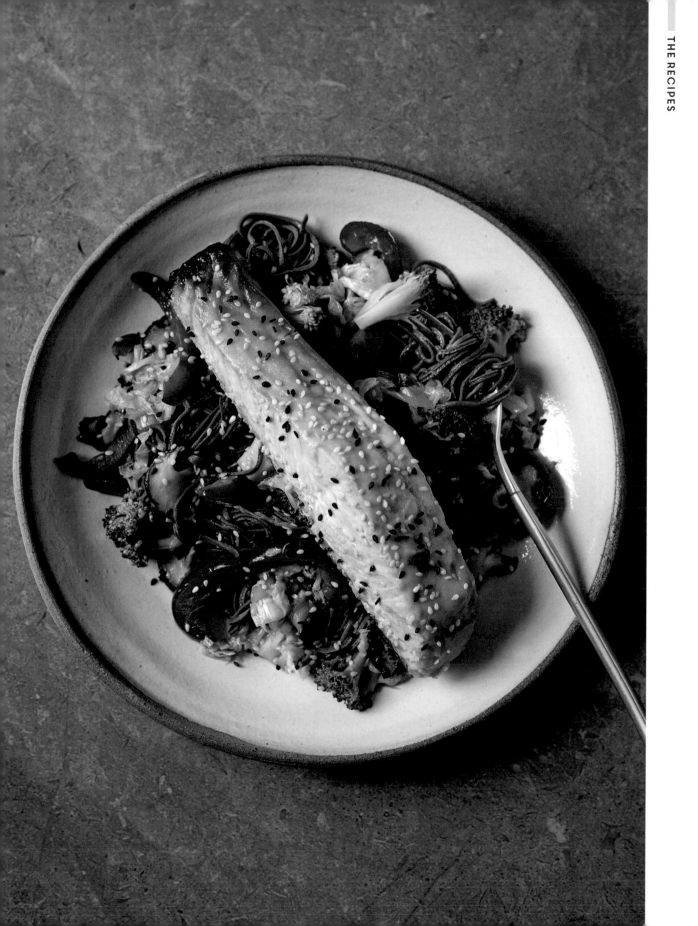

SERVES 4

Holy guacamole! This dip works brilliantly with crudités, such as carrot sticks, celery strips and red pepper batons. It's also a great healthy party food. If you want it to look extra pretty, garnish it with some sliced red radishes.

GUACAMOLE

2 large ripe avocados, halved
   and destoned
2 tbsp fresh lemon juice
2 small tomatoes, halved
½ shallot, peeled
½ red chilli, deseeded
15g fresh coriander leaves
sea salt and freshly ground black
   pepper

Scoop the avocado flesh into a blender, add the lemon juice and pulse for 15–20 seconds.

Add the remaining ingredients and season with salt and pepper.

Run the blender for a further 10 seconds. (Be careful not to over-blend – the mixture should be chunky.)

TIP:
You need the avocados to be as ripe as possible. Also, it's better to use shallots rather than an onion as they don't overpower the avocado.

// NUTRITION PER SERVING: CALORIES 176 / FAT 15G / CARBS 13G / PROTEIN 3G

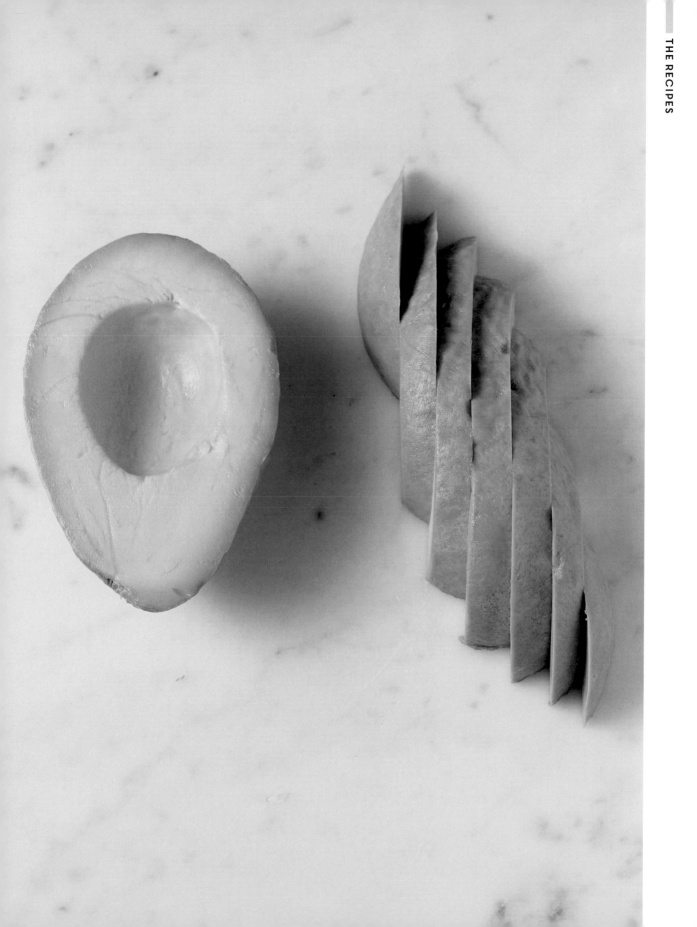

SERVES 1

This beats the shop-bought stuff, hands down. Pulses like chickpeas are full of fibre, which is good for digestion - it helps keep things regular . . . Houmous is also something you might like to experiment with. You can throw in a tin of beetroots (drained), which will make it an amazing purply pink, or a jar of peeled and roasted red peppers. Serve with crudités of your choice - try carrot batons, strips of red pepper or celery sticks. It also goes well with wholemeal pitta or wholemeal tortilla chips.

HOMEMADE HOUMOUS

1 x 660g jar chickpeas
(I recommend Brindisa
– don't use tinned)
juice of 2½ lemons
4 tbsp tahini
1 tbsp olive oil
pinch of cayenne pepper
sea salt and freshly ground black
pepper

Pop the entire contents of the jar of chickpeas including the liquid into a blender. Add the lemon juice, tahini, olive oil and cayenne, and season with salt and pepper, to taste. Whizz until the mixture is smooth.

// NUTRITION PER SERVING: CALORIES 64 / FAT 3G / CARBS 11G / PROTEIN 1G

Latkes are potato pancakes that are a Hanukkah tradition. Parsnips and carrots are not traditional ingredients, but after trying this recipe you'll wonder why you haven't used them before.

PARSNIP & CARROT LATKES

100g carrots, peeled and grated

150g Desiree potatoes, peeled and grated

200g parsnips, peeled and grated

2 medium free-range egg whites

1 tbsp gram flour

a large pinch of freshly ground black pepper

2 tbsp snipped fresh chives

60g clarified butter

1 tbsp crème fraiche

Place the carrots in a tea towel and squeeze out as much moisture as possible.

Repeat this process with the potatoes and parsnip.

Mix the egg whites, gram flour, pepper and chives together in a large bowl.

Add all the grated vegetables and mix well.

Place a frying pan over a medium to high heat and add half the butter. Take a handful of the mixture and place in the pan to form a nice round latke. Continue with more mixture, trying to fit 4 latkes in the pan at once. Cook for 2 minutes, until golden, then turn to crisp the other side. Don't allow the pan to get too hot and burn your latkes.

Remove from the heat and set aside to keep warm.

Repeat this process with the remaining mixture until all the latkes have been cooked.

Serve with a dollop of crème fraiche on top.

// NUTRITION PER LATKE: CALORIES 121 / FAT 9G / CARBS 8G / PROTEIN 2G

MAKES 40 BITES

When you crave something sweet but want to avoid refined sugar or a chocolate bar, reach for these instead. You might want to keep some in your fridge for just such an occasion - but that doesn't mean you can scoff one every day. They're still a treat!

SKINNY CHOCOLATE BROWNIES

250g cashew nuts

130g cocoa powder

250g Medjool dates, pitted

1 tbsp coconut oil, melted and cooled

130g pecan nuts, halved

Line a 30 x 20cm baking tray with baking paper.

Put the cashew nuts into a blender and whizz for 30 seconds, until they start to look a bit like sand. Make sure you don't overdo it, as the oil will begin to separate.

Add the cocoa powder and pulse on and off for about 1 minute.

Add the dates and coconut oil and blend for 2−3 minutes, until smooth.

Spoon into a bowl and use a wooden spoon or spatula to mix in the pecan nuts.

Turn into the tray and level the top – it should be around 1cm thickness.

Place in the fridge for 20 minutes, or until solid.

Cut up and enjoy!

// NUTRITION PER SERVING: CALORIES 141 / FAT 12G / CARBS 10G / PROTEIN 4G

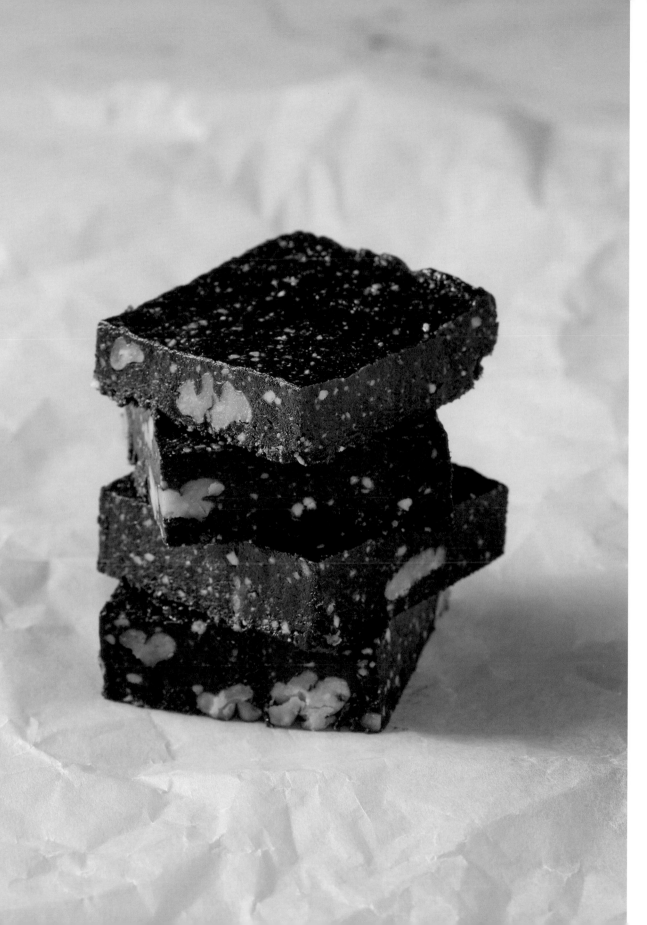

SERVES 1

Hell, yes, you can have a sweet treat! This shake is the
perfect mix between salty and sweet – just minus the sugar
and minus the guilt.

SALTED CARAMEL DATE SHAKE

2 Medjool dates, pitted
180ml almond milk
1 tsp vanilla extract
½ tsp sea salt
½ tsp lemon juice
8 ice cubes

Place all the ingredients in a blender and whizz on high speed
until you have a smooth consistency.

Drink immediately.

// NUTRITION PER SERVING: CALORIES 189 / FAT 2G / CARBS 64G / PROTEIN 2G

MAKES 2 PORTIONS

Did you know that bananas are the food item most likely to be thrown away? Shoppers in Britain throw away 1.4 million edible bananas every day. I get it: there's a short window when they switch from perfectly ripe to mush, but that doesn't mean you need to bin them. Instead, as they start to go brown, chop them into chunks and freeze them. Then, when you fancy a quick snack, pop them into the blender with some nut milk and, hey presto, banana ice cream! You can throw in some frozen strawberries, too, to change it up.

CHEAT'S BANANA ICE CREAM

4 bananas, sliced
25ml almond milk

Freeze the bananas for 4–6 hours or overnight.

Place the frozen banana slices in a blender with the almond milk and whizz for 2 minutes.

// NUTRITION PER SERVING: CALORIES 245 / FAT 1G / CARBS 60G / PROTEIN 2G

MAKES 10 PORTIONS

Want to go vegan but fear you'll miss proper chocolate too much? Try this. It's not just butter and milk free - it is also sugar free. The bark is easy to make and hits the spot when you need a sweet treat.

DAIRY-FREE WHITE CHOCOLATE BARK

150g cacao butter

120g cashew butter

60g agave nectar

40g dried cranberries, roughly chopped

40g dried apricots, roughly chopped

½ vanilla pod, split and deseeded

60g roasted cashews, roughly chopped

40g pistachio nuts, shelled and roughly chopped

Line a large 30 x 38cm baking tray with baking paper.

Place the cacao butter in a bowl and place the bowl over a saucepan of simmering water. Gently melt the butter, stirring constantly, making sure not to burn it.

Take the bowl off the heat once the butter is completely melted and whisk in the cashew butter and agave nectar.

Stir in the cranberries, apricots and the seeds from the vanilla pod.

Once everything is combined, pour on to the prepared baking tray and scatter over the cashews and pistachios.

Refrigerate for 6 hours or overnight.

Once set, break into pieces and store in an airtight container in the fridge for up to 10 days – if you can resist.

Tuck in and enjoy!

// NUTRITION PER 50G SERVING: CALORIES 300 / FAT 27G / CARBS 17G / PROTEIN 3G

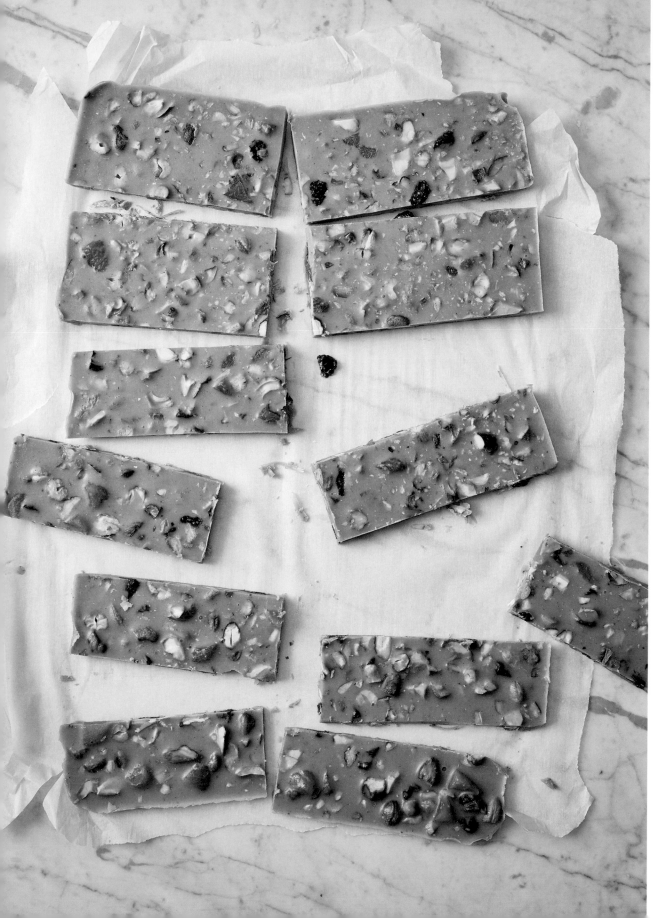

MAKES 4 PORTIONS

Tamagoyaki are Japanese rolled omelettes - usually served in a bento box as a side dish or eaten for breakfast.

JAPANESE PAN-FRIED EGG ROLLS AKA TAMAGOYAKI

4 medium free-range eggs

1 tsp rapeseed oil, plus extra
   for greasing

¼ tsp salt

¼ tsp soy sauce

1 tbsp mirin

Whisk the ingredients together in a large bowl.

Place a wide, non-stick frying pan over a medium to high heat and coat lightly in oil.

Pour a thin layer of the egg mixture into the pan, tilting to cover the whole pan like a pancake. When the egg has set a little, gently roll into a log – it's surprisingly easy to do this with chopsticks.

Keep the rolled log on the edge of your pan and add more egg mixture, swirling like a pancake again.

When the bottom of the egg has set and there is still liquid on top, position the first pancake at the edge and roll the new pancake over the first.

Keep adding egg to the pan and rolling back and forth until all the egg mixture is used up.

Remove the multi-layered log from the pan and place on a piece of cling film.

Tightly wrap in the cling film and cool in the fridge.

When you are ready to serve, simply cut yourself a slice – you should see a nice spiral pattern in the cross-section of the egg.

// **NUTRITION PER SERVING: CALORIES 76 / FAT 5G / CARBS 2G / PROTEIN 5G**

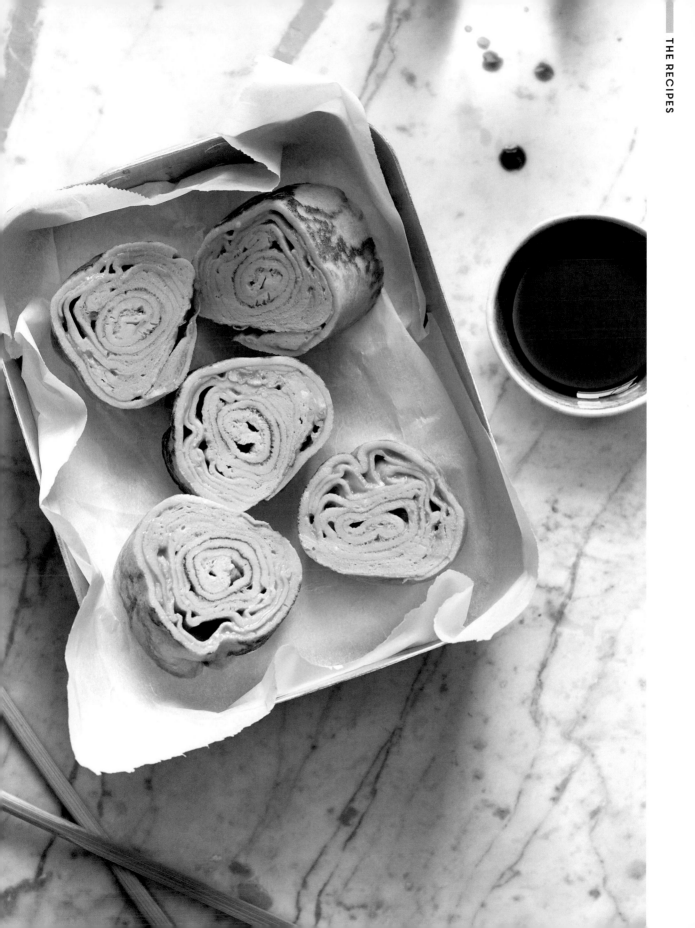

MAKES 6 PORTIONS

Not all chocolate is created equal. Don't assume that it is a food you have to avoid when you're on a health kick – dark chocolate is packed with antioxidants. In fact, dark chocolate has to be the most popular ingredient ever to win the title 'superfood'. Chocolate and avocado is a popular Aussie combo – don't knock it until you try it!

AVOCADO & DARK CHOCOLATE CHIP ICE CREAM

2 large ripe avocados, peeled, destoned and chopped
250ml coconut milk
60ml honey
60ml cocoa powder
2 tsp vanilla extract
pinch of sea salt
70g dark chocolate chips

Place all the ingredients, apart from the chocolate chips, in a blender and whizz until smooth and creamy.

Stir through the chocolate chips.

Spoon into a container and place in the freezer.

After 1 hour, whisk or mash thoroughly with a fork to break up the ice crystals and keep a smooth texture. Repeat this process 6 times, every 20–30 minutes, before finally freezing for 4–6 hours or overnight.

// NUTRITION PER SERVING: CALORIES 400 / FAT 29G / CARBS 36G / PROTEIN 5G

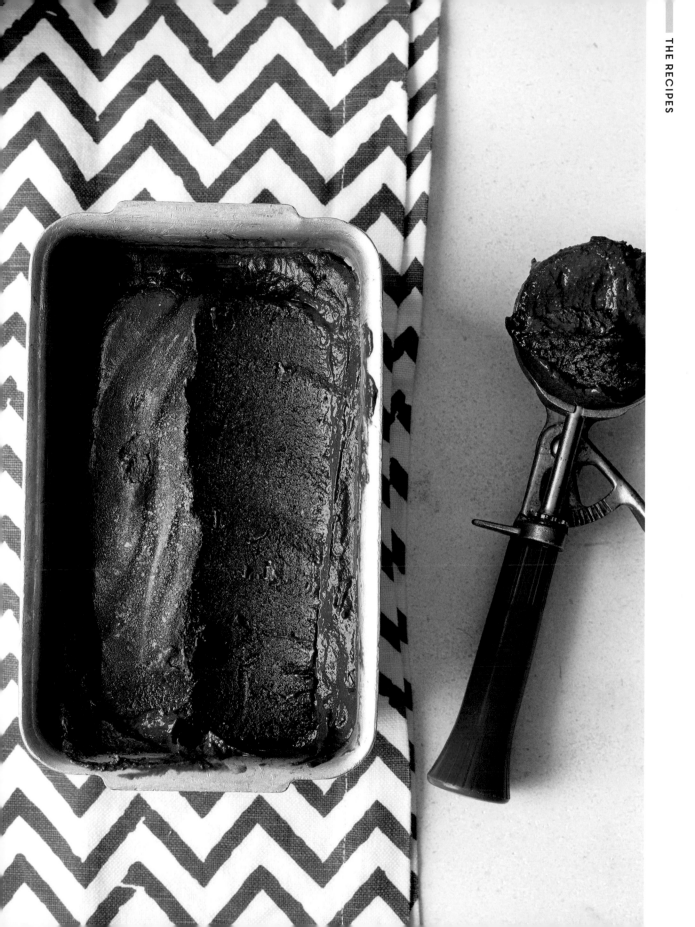

MAKES 24

Coconut always makes me think of the tropics. These energy balls are vegan and have no added sugar but they are so sweet, you may find the children raiding them . . .

APRICOT & COCONUT BALLS

150g blanched almonds
250g dried apricots
½ tsp vanilla powder
½ tsp ground cinnamon
120g desiccated coconut

Place the almonds in a blender and pulse until they start to resemble sand.

Add the apricots, vanilla powder, cinnamon and 3 tablespoons of desiccated coconut. Pulse until well mixed.

Roll the mixture into 2.5cm balls, lightly covering each ball with the remaining desiccated coconut.

Tuck in!

// NUTRITION PER BALL: CALORIES 69 / FAT 4G / CARBS 9G / PROTEIN 1G

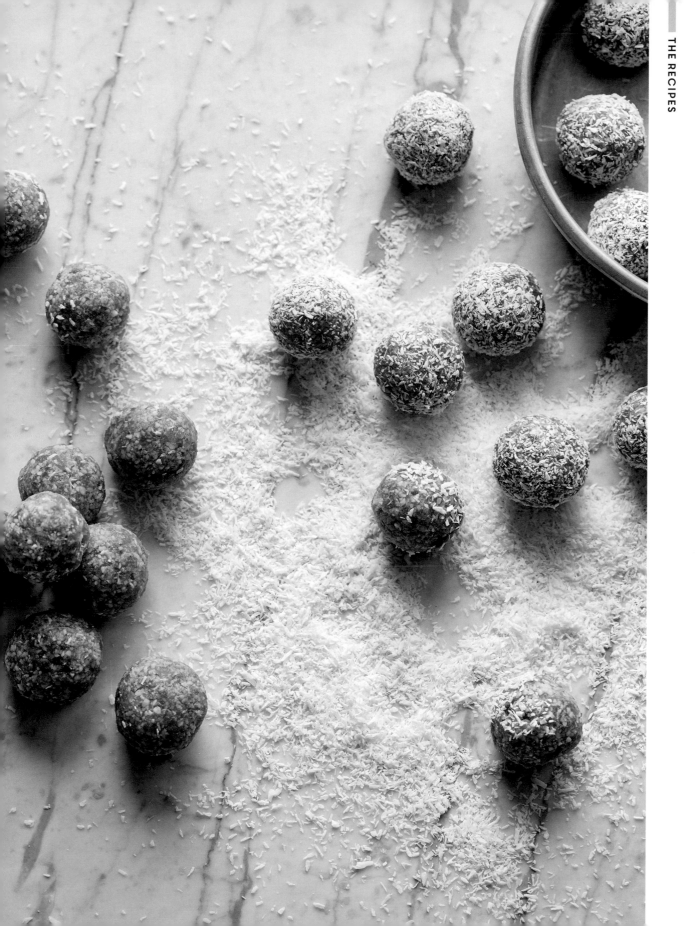

You could also **try this with chickpeas and any spice blend you like. They would go well in a salad with chicken, too.**

ROASTED SNACKING BUTTER BEANS

1 x 660g jar butter beans, drained
½ tsp dried garlic powder
1 tsp smoked paprika (mild
   or spicy, depending on your
   preference)
½ tsp celery salt
1 tsp ground cumin
2 tbsp olive oil

Preheat the oven to 180°C/Fan 160°C and line a baking tray with baking paper.

Mix all the ingredients together in a large bowl.

Pour the beans on to the baking tray and place in the oven.

Cook for 15 minutes, then shake the tray to turn the beans.

Roast for a further 15 minutes, or until nicely coloured and crisp on the outside.

// NUTRITION PER 50G SERVING: CALORIES 96 / FAT 1G / CARBS 16G / PROTEIN 4G

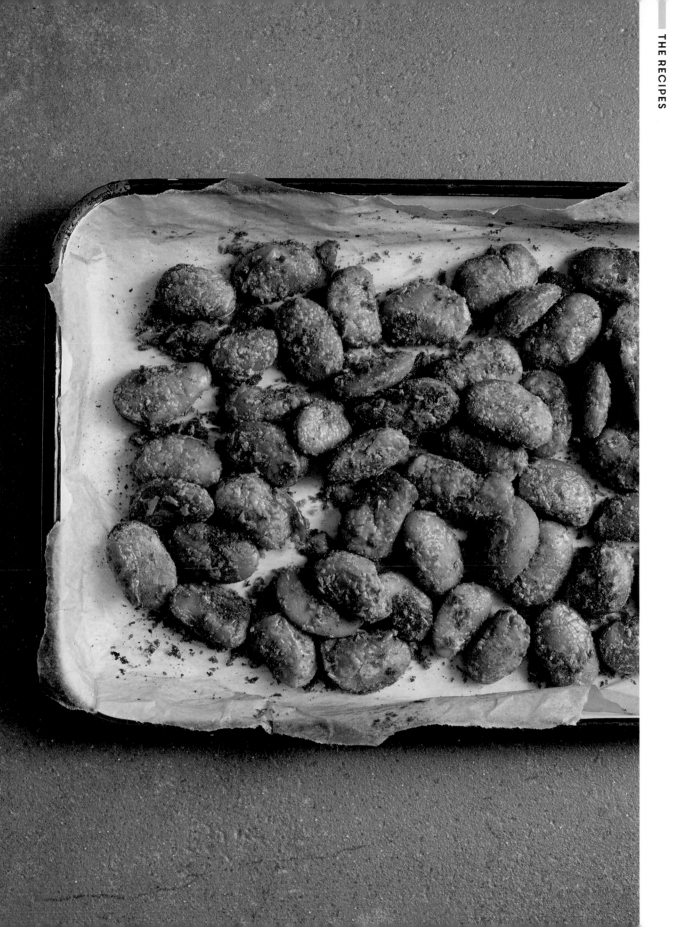

MAKES 12 BIG SLICES

Because no recipe book can be complete without some flapjacks ... These are a perfect mid-afternoon pick-me-up.

QUINOA FLAPJACKS

1 medium free-range egg white

2 tbsp molasses

3 tbsp arrowroot

1 tsp vanilla bean paste

1 tsp ground cinnamon

1 tsp bicarbonate of soda

50g butter, melted

50g ground hemp seed

360g cooked quinoa

100g mixed seeds (for example, pumpkin, sunflower and sesame)

150g desiccated coconut

75g dried fruit

1 carrot, peeled and grated

2 small apples, peeled, cored and grated

Preheat the oven to 180°C/Fan 160°C and line a 30 x 20cm baking tray with baking paper.

Mix the egg white, molasses, arrowroot, vanilla, cinnamon, bicarbonate of soda, butter and hemp seed in a large bowl. Stir until well combined.

Add the remaining ingredients.

Pour the mixture into the prepared tin and spread evenly. Bake in the oven for about 50 minutes, until golden brown.

Remove from the oven and score into 12 portions, then leave to cool.

Slice and store in an airtight container for up to 1 week.

// NUTRITION PER 1 SLICE: CALORIES 100 / FAT 8G / CARBS 13G / PROTEIN 3G

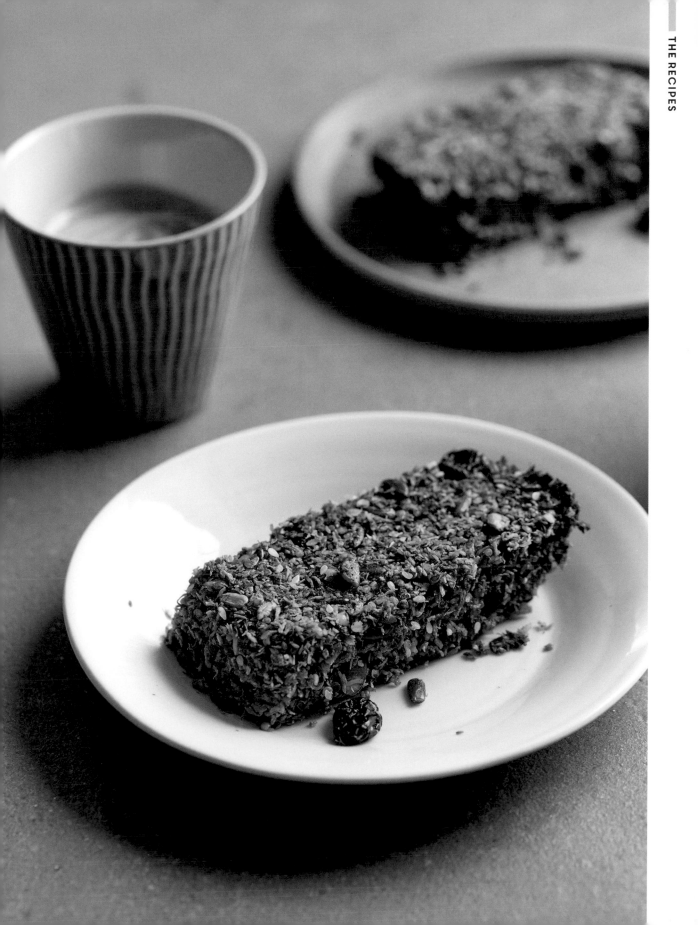

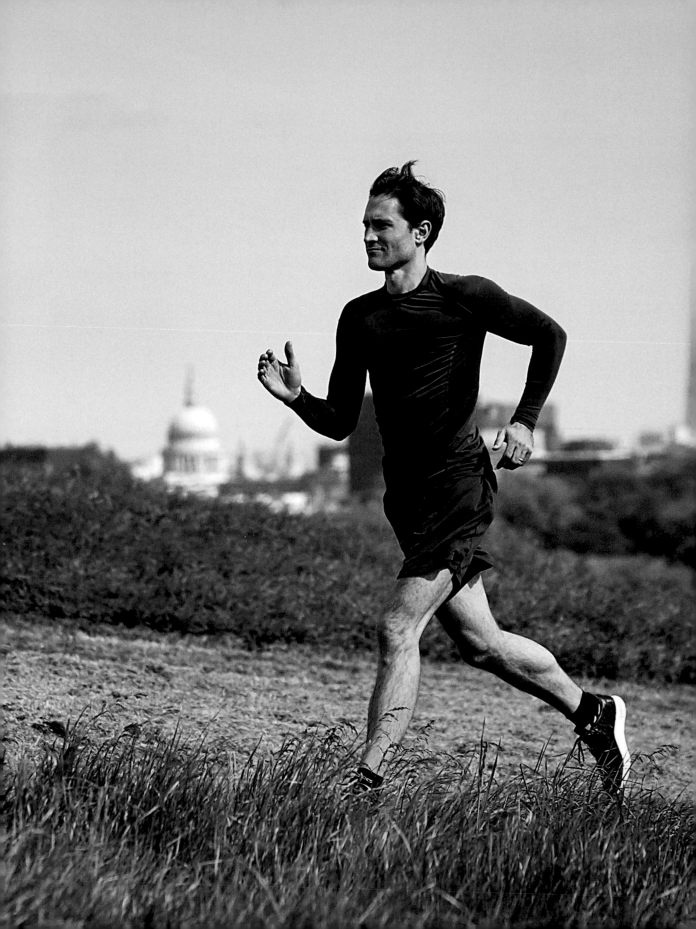

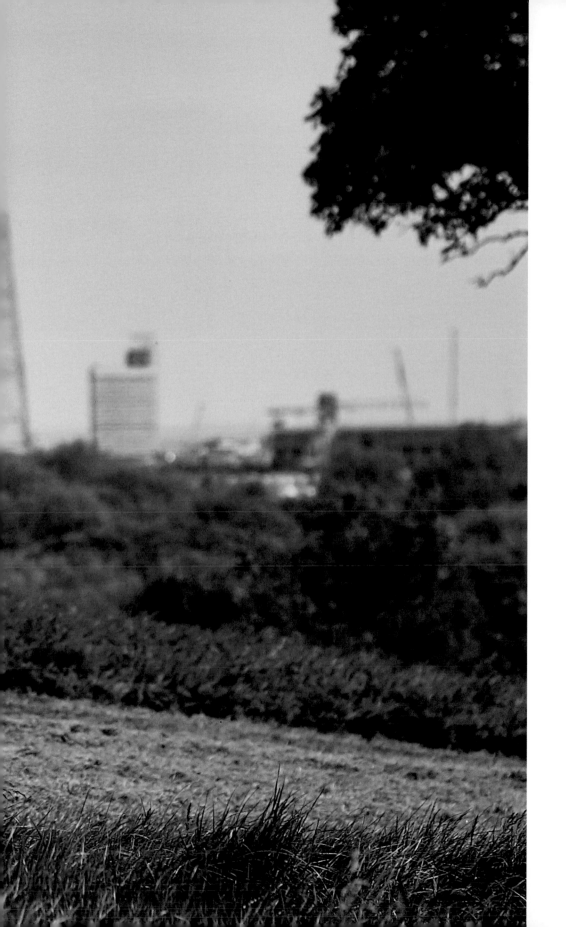

PART THREE

FOREVER FIX

BODY DYNAMIX

My Body Dynamix course is a specific prescription of exercises combined with direct stimulation of the central nervous system and together they reinforce your body's new way of moving. This is the course to turn to when you have any aches or niggles – we'll get you back on the right path as quickly as possible.

When I was studying at university, they taught us that 'Where there is pain, there is weakness.' So when I started assessing patients, I would focus on the site of the pain. As I started to learn more and practise more, however, I began using the mantra from the biochemist Ida Rolf: 'Where you think it is, it ain't.' So, if your knee hurts, focus above at the hip and below at the ankle. If your back hurts, focus on the thoracic spine and the hips. If your neck hurts, look at the skull and at the thoracic spine.

I started to look at the whole body to find the answers. For example, I've found that patients' pain and postural dysfunction generally stem from an unconscious reinforcement of poor posture due to their sedentary lifestyle, their work (sitting at a desk all day) and driving. Having once focused on the pain and the problem in isolation, now I look at the whole body.

In your body there are muscle imbalances everywhere. Most of the time we don't feel them. One day, however, you'll end up saying, 'All I did was bend over to pick up my shopping …' or my favourite, 'I have no idea what I did, I just woke up like this …'

But it's not what you just did, it's what you've been doing for the last 10, 15 or 20 years.

Our traditional approach to dealing with pain when we found it was: 'If it hurts, it's weak, so let's strengthen it with exercises' and 'If it's tight, just stretch it to make it looser.' That approach works in a small number of cases but, even then, it's guesswork. In any muscle pain/movement dysfunction there are victims (where the pain is) and culprits (sneaky muscles causing the actual problem).

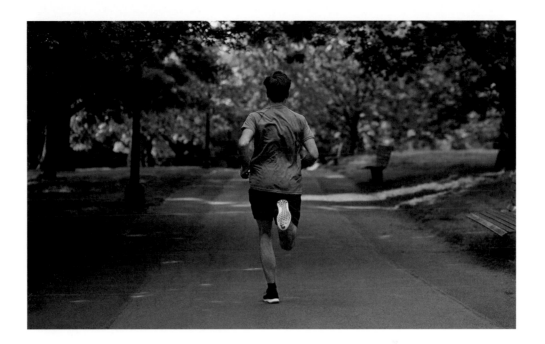

The culprits contract, forcing the victims to work against their will for far too long. But I don't blame the culprits, they're only doing their job. They are finding a way to work most efficiently in their new situation – the sedentary lifestyle.

When people want to activate a muscle that has been dormant, the most common mistake they make is to jump into it, trying to engage that muscle by doing large compound movements. But I believe to engage and recruit the right group of muscles, you must first deactivate the muscles that are opposing it or are locking it in position. So, to retract your chin, you have to turn off the tight short muscles at the front.

You can learn to disengage the opposing muscles through trigger point release. Body Dynamix is the method I use to stimulate the body's central nervous system – effectively hitting ctrl + alt + del on the entire system, allowing those overused muscles to reset and allowing the underused ones to start to do their job. It takes time to re-programme your body into a new way of moving, though. The more you do it, however, the easier and less painful everything becomes.

In order to stimulate the central nervous system, you need to use soft tissue/acupressure/myofascial release points (they're all the same) and that's why the Transformational Programme begins with a series of foam rolling.

DEEP NECK FLEXORS

NB: Don't press on anything with a pulse!

01. With the middle 3 fingers on your right hand, reach over the left side of your neck, finding the middle, just above your collar bone and below your ear lobe/ jaw bone.

02. Compress this area against the side of your vertebrae and hold for 30 seconds, remembering to feel for any tension points or pain and begin to discover that area with your fingers, manoeuvring ever so slowly.

After a minute or so locate a tender area, compress and begin to turn your head right and left while maintaining the compression on the site of pain.

03. Now, drop your right ear to your right shoulder, still maintaining the compression, and now the left ear to the left shoulder.

04. After a 2–3 minute treatment, repeat on your right side.

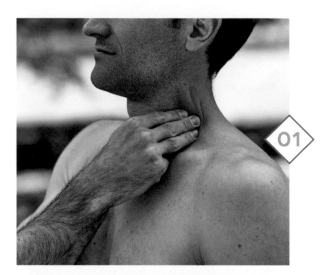

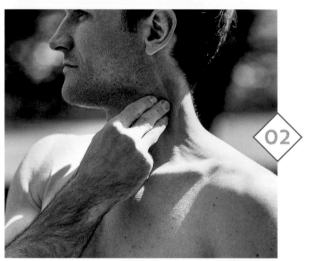

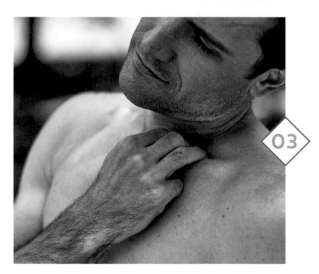

CHEST & SHOULDERS

01. Find where your left collarbone meets your breastbone. Using the first and middle fingers of your right hand, feel for the space underneath the collarbone and above your first rib.

Apply pressure into that space and begin to draw slow small circles, gradually increasing the pressure (if you can handle it) for 20 seconds.

02. Once you've found a tender area, hold the pressure for 20 seconds, then begin to rub across it, back and forth for a further 20 seconds. Remember to relax the arm and shoulder as much as possible.

03. Do this all the way until you reach your shoulder joint, then start again but this time massage between the space of your first rib and second rib. Always be on the lookout for any tender areas.

04. Do the same thing between the second and third rib.

05. Repeat on the other side.

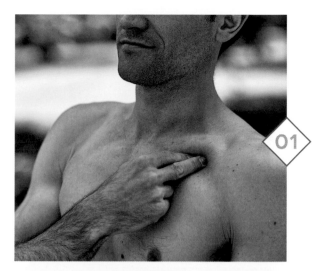

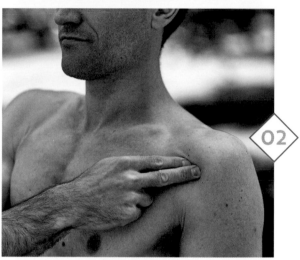

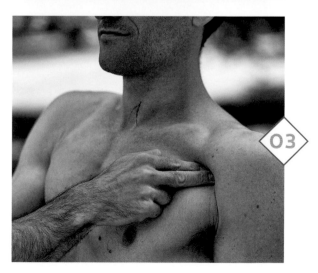

FOAM ROLLER SEQUENCE

In order to stimulate the central nervous system, you need to use soft tissue/acupressure/myofascial release points (they're all the same) and that's why the Transformational Programme begins with a series of foam rolling.

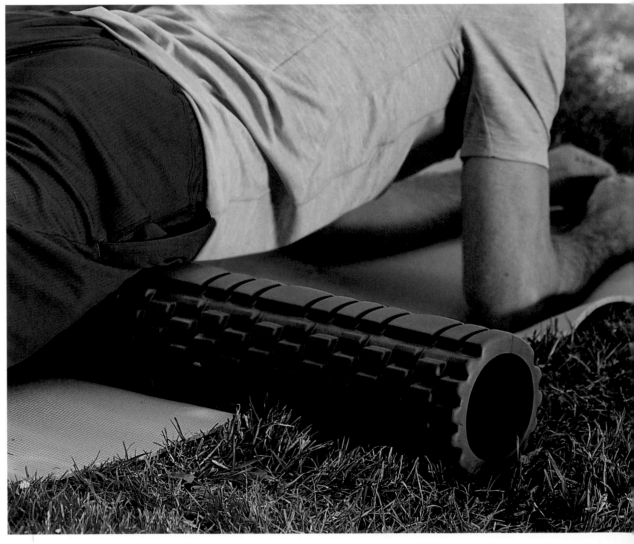

HIPS

01. Lie face down, placing the foam roller under your right thigh, just below the crest of your hip. Bend your left leg out to the side. Supporting your body weight with your forearms, slowly roll up and down or side to side on the roller until you find a tender spot. Now, hold that spot for 30 seconds and breathe, actively trying to take out all the 'protective' tension within that muscle.

02. After the initial 30 seconds, bend the right knee up behind you and slowly lengthen it back down again. Once the leg is fully extended, tense that leg by holding it straight. This will activate the muscles that the roller is pressing into. Hold it for 5 seconds then relax, consciously letting go of all the muscle tension in that area.

03. Now find another tender area around that hip complex and repeat the process of active tensing and active release all the way down the thigh, stopping just above the knee.

04. Repeat on the other side.

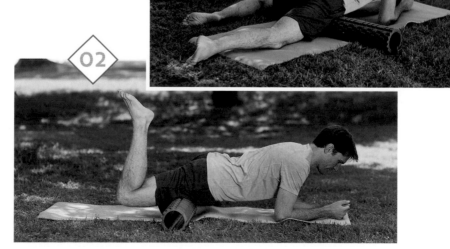

CALVES

01. Sit with the roller under your left calf. Place the palms of your hands on the ground behind your hips. Cross your right foot over the left.

02. Supporting your body weight on your hands, roll up and down the calf muscle a few times, feeling for any tight or painful areas. Once you find a tender spot, hold it for 30 seconds (dropping your hips to the floor if you can't hold yourself up).

03. Point the left toes, and then flex the foot 5 times. Hold it for 5 seconds then relax it, consciously letting go of all the muscle tension in that area.

04. Now find another tender area in the calf and repeat.

05. Repeat on the other side.

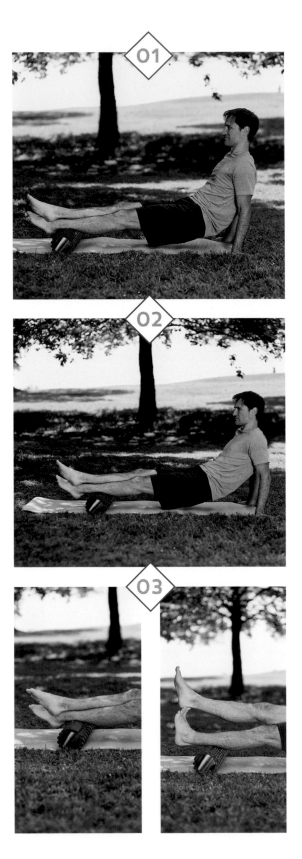

GLUTE MUSCLES

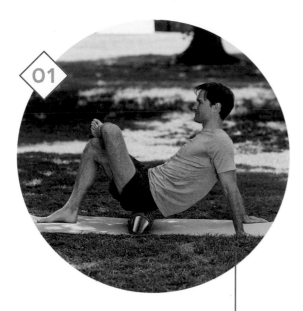

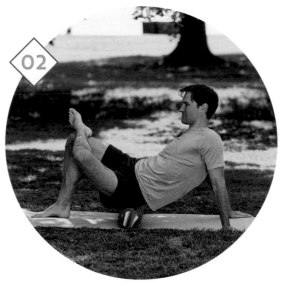

Place both hands on the floor behind you for support.

01. Sit on the edge of the foam roller, with the end of it under your left butt cheek. Bend your right knee and rest your left foot on your right knee.

02. Roll over your left glute muscles until you find a sore spot. Now, tense the left glute by actively pushing your left knee away from you.

03. After 5 seconds gently release the tension, sinking deeper into that area, and repeat until the pain subsides or for a maximum of 30 seconds.

04. Now find another tender area and repeat the process of active tensing and active release.

05. Repeat on the other side.

237

THIGHS

01. Lie on your left side with the foam roller just below your hip bone. Extend your left leg straight out, bend your right leg and place it in front of your left leg.

02. Place your left elbow and forearm on the floor for balance, and roll along your left thigh until you find a sore spot. Straighten and tense your entire leg, holding for 5 seconds then slowly relax everything, sinking deeper into the area.

Repeat until the pain subsides or for a maximum of 30 seconds.

03. Find another tender area and repeat the process of active tensing and active release until the roller is just above your knee.

04. Repeat on the other side.

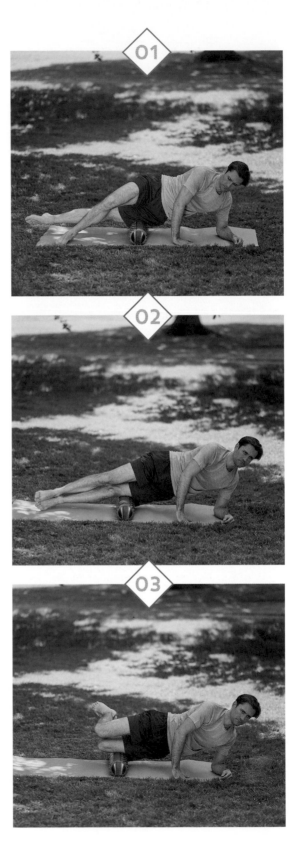

UPPER, MID & LOWER BACK

01. Position yourself on the mat with the foam roller underneath your back just below your shoulder blades, your knees bent and your feet flat on the floor. Interlock your fingers behind your head, consciously resting the muscles in the front of your neck.

Slowly lean back (remember: breathe small shallow breaths), extending all the way back as low as you can go.

02. At the bottom of the movement, breathe in. As you lift up using your abs – crunching back up again – breathe out. Repeat slowly.

03. Change the position of the roller by pushing from your feet, lifting your bum off the ground and rolling it a few inches down your back. Repeat the slow lowering of the trunk, extending over the roller, breathing in as you reach the bottom and out as you flex forward, returning to the start position once again.

04. Continue this process one vertebra at a time until you reach the top of your pelvis.

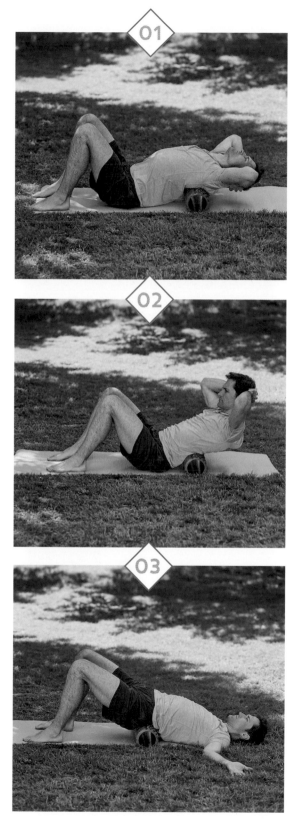

SHOULDERS

01. Lie on your left side with the roller underneath you. Support your head with your left hand. Cross your right leg over your left. Roll yourself slowly over the foam roller until the roller reaches your armpit.

02. Once the roller is at your armpit, lengthen your left hand, touching the left corner of the mat with the palm of your hand facing up. Slowly lift and move your left arm to the opposite corner of the mat and rest for a second before returning to your original position.

03. Repeat 20 times.

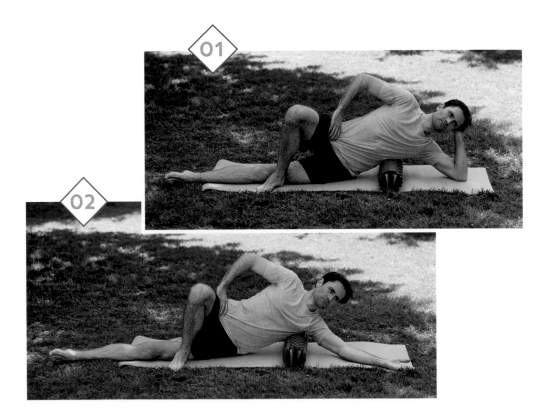

FEET

NB: You need a tennis ball or something a similar size and shape.

01. While standing (or sitting if you have to) roll the ball between your foot and the floor. Work slowly, searching for pain points.

02. Once you find a pain point, hold the pressure on it for 20 seconds.

03. Without changing position, slowly work the ball left and right of the area while maintaining the pressure (or increasing the pressure if you feel you can handle it).

04. Move on and find any other areas of pain.

05. Repeat on the other foot.

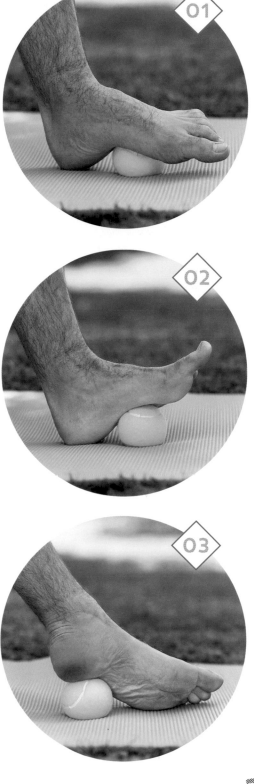

SIMPLE TRICKS
FOR STICKING WITH
THE PROGRAMME

Losing weight and getting fitter isn't really about the body, it's about the mind. How can you ensure the changes you make are successful? To change your behaviour, you have to change the situation around you – your environment. That means having the right healthy foods in the fridge and avoiding fast food joints.

There are things even more important than your environment that you need to change – your heart and your mind. So what happens when the heart wants something and the brain wants something else? It's really two parts of your brain in competition with each other. The rational side – looking towards the future – wants you to forgo the pack of biscuits, but the emotional side wants the immediate pleasure of eating that biscuit.

The relationship you're going to have with food and your body is like a good relationship with a romantic partner. You need both your heart and your head to tell you it is a good match if you want it to work out. The head will say, 'You need to eat more vegetables, stop eating so much sugar and get moving everyday.' But if your heart's not invested in it – there's no 'why' – then what's the point? On the other hand, if you're all heart and no brain, then there's no plan behind your drive. 'I'm going to get super motivated and pumped up, and we'll just go crazy at it.'

The heart is easier to win over. That's when you're thinking, 'I want to change.' You've bought this book, so we already know your heart is in it. But support comes with the method, the programme and the online community (David Higgins London community Facebook page) I'm building to back you up.

There will be moments when this programme will feel hard. You'll probably know your own weaknesses from past attempts to lose weight, get fit and improve your health. Maybe it's when you have one biscuit and you think, 'I've broken my diet now, I might as well finish off the packet.' Or perhaps you find yourself too overwhelmed at work to exercise or think about what you're eating. That's why it is vital to lay good foundations in the first 21 days to build on later. You have put yourself on a new path, now you need to stay on it. Here's how:

BE YOUR OWN CHEERLEADER

Celebrate and recognise what you are doing – you are transforming. You should also keep returning to the commitment you wrote on day one (see page 18) – read it for inspiration if you are ever tempted to give up. But also read it when you've eaten a slice of cake against your better judgement and are mulling over whether to have a second. There's no shame in occasionally indulging; what is important is that you don't then sabotage yourself by having a mega blowout.

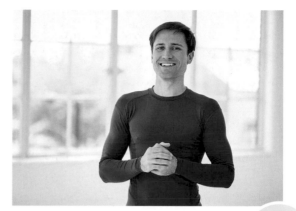

BE CONSISTENT

Consistency is key – aim to exercise at the same time each day, for example. This won't always be possible, but it should be a goal. It means you are finding time for yourself.

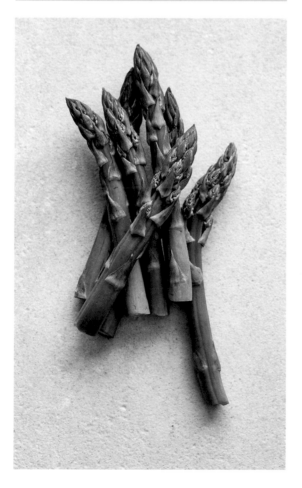

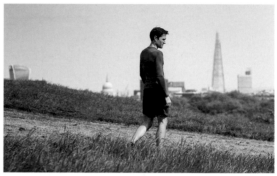

DON'T OBSESS ABOUT THE NUMBER ON THE SCALES

Do track your weight, but not obsessively. If you weigh yourself daily, you are likely to spot natural fluctuations – such as when women are pre-menstrual or if you've drunk a lot of water. This can be demoralising. It is much better that you take a longer-term approach to weight-watching. A weekly weigh-in will be more useful to you.

THE PSYCHOLOGICAL PRINCIPLES OF HABIT-FORMING

The world around us doesn't make it easy to stay thin. There are temptations all around: the confectionery aisle, the cupcake shop, the biscuit tin. At the end of the 21-day Body Reset Programme, I don't expect every one of my readers never to eat a biscuit again but what I do hope is that you'll have control over when you really want that biscuit and when you're happy saying 'no'. And I want you to be able to say 'yes' to one, but 'no' to finishing off the packet.

Magazines, books and TV shows usually peddle quick fixes, promising dramatic weight loss, but if you think how long it took you to gain the weight, you'll realise that it will take time to lose it. Try not to see that as a problem. If you lose the weight in a slow, controlled way and you change the environment around you, rather than thinking of weight loss as a period of deprivation followed by a return to your old habits, you are much more likely to keep the weight off. It takes time to turn new behaviours into healthier habits but, once they are habits, they will keep you on the right path.

One of the biggest problems with diets is the word itself. Think about what the word means to you – you'll think of deprivation, feeling hungry, feeling miserable and going without what you enjoy. And willpower is finite. For everyone. Think of it as a muscle. Every time you use it, you tire it, and you are less able to use it again. So, resisting food over and over again is mentally exhausting. It drains you.

Supervising ourselves takes it out of you. We run on auto-pilot a lot of the time; changing behaviour forces you to take control. You need to understand this to change your behaviour with health and exercise. A lot of your behaviour will have become automatic. You're not really thinking it through.

TIPS

01/
MINDFUL EATING

We often joke about 'eating our feelings'. What we mean is comfort eating – the way we turn to certain calorific foods when we're feeling blue (as epitomised by Bridget Jones eating ice cream in her PJs). This is a very easy trap to fall into. But what it really represents is mindless eating. So, when you're next tempted, ask yourself these simple questions:

A. Why am I eating this?

B. Will it make me feel better or worse in an hour's time?

If the answer to (a) is 'To make myself feel better' and the answer to (b) is 'Worse', you can see there's a contradiction. Now you can see there's no logic to it, choose something else that will genuinely make you feel better – have a hot bubble bath, go for a walk, do some stretches, or call a friend.

02/
PLAN AHEAD

If you know that you overeat when you go out to restaurants, look at the menu online and pick your food in advance. That will stop you straying towards the unhealthy dishes.

03/
BE KIND TO YOURSELF

Overeating is often linked to self-criticism. You tell yourself, 'I'm hopeless,' chipping away at your confidence, and that drives you towards unhealthy food. Instead, be your biggest cheerleader. Don't feel any shame in saying, 'I'm brilliant' and 'I deserve better than to put myself down.' You *are* brilliant!

04/
TACKLE YOUR TRIGGERS

Perhaps you always overeat when you go to the cinema; you've come to associate the cinema with a big bucket of popcorn. You need to break this pattern. Start by bringing a healthy snack of your own – my Skinny Chocolate Brownies (see page 212), for example. That way you still have a treat but you don't overeat.

05/
TACKLE YOUR TRIGGER TIMES

It isn't just certain events that lead us to overeat but certain times of the day, too. I know so many people whose first reaction on getting home is to open the fridge. Make a new getting-home-from-work ritual: go and sit in the garden in the summer, or take half an hour to yourself to read a book in the winter.

HOW TO SUPPORT SOMEONE ON THE PROGRAMME

If you are following my programme but your significant other isn't, this is the section to hand to them. It's also helpful for friends and family to read.

ENCOURAGEMENT

So, your partner, friend or family member has decided to change their life – be impressed by their resolve! But in the same spirit as 'It takes a village to raise a child', it usually takes a team to help someone lose weight and get fitter. If you have never struggled with your weight, it can be hard to grasp why others find weight loss so hard. So the most important message for you is to listen. Find out what they are trying to achieve so you can work out how best to support them.

At the right time, ask (gently!) what their barriers to getting fit have been in the past, or the factors that have contributed to their weight gain. Then think about what you can do to mitigate those problems and offer not just emotional support but practical assistance. You need to help change the environment around them to make it easier for them to succeed.

Perhaps stress has been a barrier in the past. When their job gets busy, they start rewarding themselves with sugary treats and find they've got no time to exercise. This is where you can help. Think of ways you can remove stresses from their life.

It's really important to be careful with your tone when you talk about their weight, though. Don't be patronising: no one likes being lectured. Never nag. It's OK to check in with them, but don't sound like you're checking up on them. The worst approach is to make them feel guilt or shame about what they put in their mouths. This can encourage secret eating. Be patient, too.

They may complain that they are not losing weight fast enough – remind them that sustainable weight loss isn't about instant results – losing weight slowly and keeping that weight off is far better than yo-yo dieting. But when they have lost weight, notice. Losing weight is a psychological battle. When people feel they are already part of the way there, they are more likely to stick with the rest of the programme. People need to think they are making progress, because it's easy to become demoralised. Remember this and focus on the positive changes they've already made.

But be supportive if they do slip up. Never focus on mistakes. A day off the programme isn't a disaster. If they've fallen off the horse, be the one who gives them a leg-up to get back on.

FOOD

Clear the cupboard of trigger items – chocolate, crisps, sweets or cakes. Learn to prepare healthy food yourself. It's expensive, time-intensive and stressful to make separate meals so be willing to eat better yourself. Eating more vegetables and less junk food benefits us all, even if you don't need or want to lose weight.

When you're eating out, pick a restaurant where there are healthy options. When you're going somewhere where it will be hard to stick to the programme (a weekend away with friends, say), plan strategies to help them cope.

Don't ever tempt someone to stray from the programme. You are being a diet saboteur. It might come from a place of insecurity on your part (in which case, think about why that is) but it certainly won't serve them well.

Finally, remember that many people use food as an emotional crutch. If you can offer support so they talk to you when they're down or stressed, you may find that they are less likely to turn to food for comfort.

EXERCISE

Couples who work (out) together, stay together. OK, so I made that up, but shared experiences tighten the bonds between us and our partners and friends. There is no reason why you shouldn't do the 21-day Body Reset Programme together. It will benefit your neck, back and core especially.

Try to fit more movement into the day. When you're together, walk up escalators and take the stairs instead of the lift. If you often spend evenings slumped in front of the TV, go to a Pilates class together instead or just out for a walk. Make 'date night' (if you do it) fitness-focused. Try a dance class instead of going out drinking (alcohol is high in calories).

247

WHAT NOT TO SAY

'You just need to eat less and move more. How hard can that be?'

That isn't supportive or kind and yet people do still say it, even to their nearest and dearest.

'It's easy - just do this . . .'

This will come across as patronising. What worked for you might not be right for them. Weight loss and getting fit are individual – you might swear by an app that tracks how many calories you've eaten, but that may be your partner's idea of torture. It's also not a great approach to offer unsolicited advice, or to paint yourself as a role model for your partner.

'You're always at the gym; what about me?'

Unless they really are spending every waking hour there, saying this makes you a diet saboteur. Could you exercise with them instead?

'Oh, go on, one biscuit won't hurt.'

'You're not fat. You don't need to diet.'

This is a common one. Sounds loving, doesn't it? Whether your partner is overweight or not, they don't need you to undermine their attempts to start eating more healthily. (There's an important exception here: if you genuinely believe they have disordered eating.)

Anything that could be construed as nagging.

You should be on your other half's team. Be their biggest cheerleader, not their biggest critic. It is very lonely to be in a relationship when you feel you're being chipped away at by incessant nagging.

WHAT TO SAY

'Don't fixate on the scales, focus on how you feel.'

'What can I do to make this easier for you?'

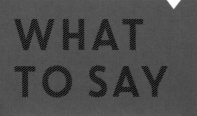

Give compliments.

This should be the easy part. Everyone likes to hear they look great.

'How can I help?'

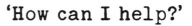

'Why don't we go for a walk instead?'

See, even
I have bad
habits I
need to be
mindful of!

CONCLUSION

Give yourself a massive pat on the back. I hope the fact that you're reading this means you have done the exercises, made many of the recipes and you're feeling much better in yourself now (I'm guessing you haven't just flicked to the back to see how it ends . . .). You are a superstar – take a moment to feel proud of yourself and what you've achieved.

There's a famous quote: **'The distance is nothing; it's only the first step that is difficult.'**

That, unfortunately, isn't true with exercise. So a thousand well dones for all the changes you've made in the past 16 weeks.

You should now be holding yourself better; moving better; resting better – simply existing better. Doing the *Hollywood Body Plan* will have put you on a new path, one that has taken you and your body in the opposite direction to where you were heading before. Hopefully, you're incorporating everything you have learned into your regular life. You now know both quick fixes and a longer-term strategy to get your body working at its best, free from pain.

To maintain the advantages of the plan, I would recommend that you keep doing the Transformational Programme 3–4 times per week. And if you do fall off the wagon – you've become busy at work or with the kids and that's taken its toll on you – always remember that you can return to the full plan again. You now know both that it works and that you can do it.

Be kind to yourself. Remember that taking time for self-care – to exercise; to cook a healthy meal – isn't selfish at all. You are the protagonist in your own story and you deserve to feel the very best you can. I'm just glad you let me come on this journey with you.

ACKNOWLEDGEMENTS

I must start by thanking my wife Cara. You saw the potential in the Aussie guy at the gym and agreed to come on this journey with me. You are the one who taught me how to breathe. The greatest gift you gave me is our 3 amazing sons, who make me feel like a Hollywood star whenever I walk through the door. Everything I do is for you all.

My Australian family, Mum and Dad: You said I could achieve anything if I set my mind to it and you gave me the freedom to try. You made a house full of boys so much fun and now I follow your blueprint with my own sons. Thank you for your love, guidance and patience.

My English family, The Hauptmans: You took me into your family with open arms and treated me like one of your own from the very beginning. Thank you.

The real superheroes here are my writing partner Ros, agent Charlie and all the team at Headline publishing, especially Muna and Kate, the designers Nikki Dupin and Emma Wells from Studio nic&lou and photographer Andrew Burton. If it wasn't for all of your hard work, dedication and encouragement, this book would never have happened.

Finally, to those of you who prove on the big screen that my method works, Sam, Margs, the director, the supermodel, the cook, the secret agent, the Amazonian, the handsome one, #borglife, a witch, a wizard and my personal editor who is the one person who has probably read this more times than me.

INDEX

RECIPE INDEX